Unleash Your True
Athletic Potential

Julianne Soviero

ISBN-10: 0692273034
ISBN-13: 978-0692273036 (Type A Publishing)

DEDICATION

To all of the athletes, performers, and fitness-lovers out there who need the information in this book to reach the next level. This book was made to help you achieve your dreams. Get ready to amaze.

CONTENTS

ACKNOWLEDGMENTS

I have so many people to thank and am so incredibly grateful for all of the wonderful people who surround me. This book would not have been possible without the support of my parents, whose influence is beyond words. My brother, an amazing writer and a creative genius, helps me edit, brainstorm and generally try to be better than him (just kidding, Jim: you are a way better writer than me). My husband is my biggest cheerleader, a great source of practical advice on editing, and a person with whom I am incredibly lucky to share my life.

This book literally would not have existed without the urging of Rob Crews (creator of A-Game), who called my unwillingness to write a whole book about athletic performance "being selfish." Thank you for getting me in gear, Rob!

I am forever grateful to Kristina Strobel, one of the most amazing photographers on the face of the planet and the creator of the stunning cover for this book. She is also my best friend and a huge inspiration to me. She always convinces me to reach higher and think bigger. View more of her unbelievable work at http://www.kristinastrobel.com.

I am so thankful for all of the amazing doctors, trainers, physical therapists, acupuncturists, and coaches who have shared their knowledge with me so that I could create this book. Dr. Christie Harrington, Madeline Martinez, Dr. Jim Masone and Dr. Donald Wallace have all shaped the way I view injury recovery and health. I would never have been able to pitch again were it not for the tireless efforts of amazing physical therapist Dr. Jeff Corben (owner of Central Sports Care), Dr. Steven Lee, and Dr. Ken Kalman. Jeff has also answered a lot of questions for me about the best training techniques. He and Dr. Stephen Nicholas made the publication of our study on the "Performance Demand of Softball Pitching" possible.

Many thanks to Brandon Marcello of Stanford University for letting me shadow him for a whole week and pick his brilliant brain.

I wouldn't have gotten very far as a softball player without the support and guidance of the Edwards family and Hofstra University. Kaci Clark,

Danielle Henderson, and Chris Aigotti have all been amazing athletes whom I have had the pleasure of looking up to and learning from.

I wouldn't have been able to get my business off of the ground without the guidance and help of Deanna Dovak, who walked me through all of the headaches involved with getting permits, insurance and so on. I still bother her all of the time with business questions.

A huge "thank you" to Dean, Noel and Sara, who introduced the idea of a plant-based diet and gave lots of great advice about it. This way of eating and living has clearly changed my life forever.

Thank you to Susan Eckert, who made me look and feel beautiful. You are an artist! Thank you to Kathy Rhind, who has showed me how flexibility and focus are an integral part of true potential.

Thank you to Archie Snowden, a talented reporter and a wonderful person, who was the very first one to think that the work I am doing is newsworthy.

This book would have been nothing but a collection of words in a computer were it not for the great guidance and advice from Bradley Communications, particularly my publicity consultant, Martha Bullen. Her patience and expertise were integral in sending me in the right direction.

Finally, how could I have written this book without daily inspiration from my wonderful athletes? Thank you all for challenging me and driving my desire to learn. It is for you that I have compiled the very best information out there

CHAPTER ONE:
A STORY OF OBESSION

If you look at my list of athletic accomplishments over the years, you might think, "she must be a great athlete."

And you would be wrong.

I am definitely a *dedicated* athlete. I commit myself to learning everything possible about any sport I choose to participate in. Then I practice until I can do the movements required of me somewhat adequately.

Then I practice more.

But, if you want to know the truth, I am not one of those people who can just magically do any sport well. I am tall and clumsy in a way that only other pitchers (and sometimes catchers) understand. I am not in any way like a graceful, stalking cheetah. I am more like a pelican: kind of awkward while walking around, but fluid in flight. My pitching coach used to say that I would have a lot of trouble walking and chewing gum at the same time, but I thrive in competition.

When I first started in competitive sports, I practiced because I was abysmal at pitching but wanted nothing more than to be a starter. I didn't have any of the things that a starting pitcher should have had: I was not fast, accurate or even particularly intimidating. I knew that practice was the only thing that I could do to stop sitting the bench all of the time. So I followed my dad all over the place with a ball and glove and he was more than happy to catch any time I asked.

He seriously chased a lot of balls. I mean, probably more than a marathon's worth.

That is probably part of the reason why, when one of my coaches suggested I go to an overnight camp at Hofstra University for a week, he enthusiastically endorsed the idea.

Let someone else go chase those balls for seven days straight!

I was personally really scared to be spending a full week away from home in a dorm where the lights only worked sometimes (and when they did they made weird buzzing sounds) and I didn't know anyone. I was only twelve at the time and I was extremely shy.

Of course, about ten minutes into the start of camp, my alleged roommate, who was eighteen and drove herself to the camp, found friends that she decided she wanted to bunk with and left me there on my own.

Awesome.

Creepy dorm: check

Lights not working properly: check

Roommate bailed: of course

So despite the fact that I kind of already hated the whole situation within the first ten minutes, I trudged through. We were assigned to two specific coaches whom we worked with all day on basic skills like hitting, fielding, base-running and throwing. All of the positional players had downtime after dinner, but us pitchers went to the football field every night to work under the lights.

And then I would go back to my creepy, empty dorm room and practice the motion into the closet door.

For the record, my first time using an alarm clock on my own was mildly disastrous, especially since I was so tired from being active all day long. Hofstra was the first time in my life when I really ate, slept and breathed a sport. Since I was under the constant supervision of some amazing coaches (several of whom later became close friends of mine), I really started to understand more about how my body moved versus how it was supposed to move, and that opened up a new world for me.

I slept fourteen hours my first day back at home.

I think mom and dad probably put a mirror over my mouth a few times to make sure I was still breathing.

Of course, making yourself better is a lot of exhausting work, and it is especially difficult if you don't know anything about recovery. I certainly didn't. Outside of camp, I was in the habit of running two miles every morning and two miles every night. I wish that I could say it was to better my performance or cross-train, but it was really because I wanted to be skinny. The unfortunate consequence of wanting to be skinny was that I had some pretty disordered eating: incidentally, one of the worst things you can possibly do for recovery.

Despite these factors, I returned to Hofstra every year and continued to progress. The first year, no one who was teaching pitching really paid me any extra attention (I noticed they really only gave lots of attention to the girls who were already pretty good), but by the second and third year, I was getting the coaches to notice. By the time I had completed my tenure at Hofstra camp I knew I would be actually playing against them the following year at Division I Manhattan College.

But all was not well in paradise. I had a decent freshman year in college, though it wasn't nearly what I was capable of. What bothered me more, though, was that I was always tired and typically in a lot of pain from practices and workouts. Not only that, but my speed and spins really seemed to have plateaued and I couldn't figure out a way around it. My sophomore year was actually much worse, as my wrist and forearm were becoming increasingly painful and kept requiring me to take time off. Eventually I did a cortisone injection, but it still did not help the pain.

Since none of the doctors could really give me a definitive reason as to why I was in pain, I just kept going and kept seeing my performance actually decline. It was the first time in my life that had ever happened and it was devastating to see so much hard work yield such bad results. I was finally diagnosed with a torn cartilage on the ulnar side of my wrist. I had been pitching with it that way for over a year. The doctor suggested

4

surgery.

So, if I knew then what I know now, my recovery from surgery would have been very different. At the time, however, I didn't want to get fat, and I couldn't get as much exercise as I would have liked with a huge cast on, hence more eating issues. I was so dumb. So, so dumb. I have no doubt whatsoever that this really slowed by body's ability to heal itself.

It wasn't until a year and half after my surgery that I could actually start to throw somewhere near the level I was at before the injury.

That is my biggest regret in sports to date.

So I lost my entire junior year and had a decent senior year, but it wasn't until the summer after my senior year that things really started happening. While working the Hofstra camp, a dream for me since I had gone there for so many years, I met the amazing Kaci Clark. Kaci made a few changes to my mechanics and encouraged me to keep working to get faster, even though I was already out of college.

So I did. And I gained about four miles an hour. That lead me to throw the hardest I had ever thrown in my life *after* college. I was thrilled but also kind of thinking: *Worst. Timing. Ever.*

This is how I became obsessed with perfect movement.

Since I was an English Education major, after learning I had these new super powers, I went on to teach English to high school students. Though

I completely adore literature and writing, I was teaching a lot of girls how to pitch after school. That schedule coupled with creating lessons and conducting extra help was very demanding. I wasn't getting a lot of sleep. I was getting sick pretty often. So when, in the middle of my first (and only) year teaching, I got an offer to go play softball professionally in Italy, I was thrilled. Since working with Kaci, I had been dreaming about pitching and playing against the best.

I was ready to quit my job right then and there and leave for Italy.

Something stopped me. Oh right, my dad. He had always been my biggest supporter in sports, but he believed that I had made a commitment to the school district and therefore had to see it through to the end of the year.

So not fair.

I took dad's advice, because, even though I knew that teaching high school wasn't for me, I didn't want to abandon the department in the middle of the year. I handed in my resignation at the end of the year. That way, they had time to fill my position and I had time to train to play in Italy the following season.

In the meantime, I figured I would start pursuing a doctorate in psychology, so that I would be able to switch careers after I was done playing.

It's funny how things work, though. I loved my doctorate course in psychology. I would think about the lesson and its applicability long after class was over. But it was really expensive and I was starting to get so many clients interested in taking pitching lessons that I decided to teach pitching on more of a full-time basis. A few months before it was time to play in Italy, I decided to coach the Italian pitchers for a few weeks instead of going to play there for several months. I had acquired so many clients through pitching lessons that I felt I would lose my newly-budding business if I went away for too long.

The team owners in Italy were very understanding and I had a great two weeks there working with the professional athletes and one of the younger leagues. I worked and lived with a pitcher from New Zealand who was really impressive.

But even though I had decided that I couldn't take all of the time off to play professionally overseas, I still wasn't done trying to achieve my personal best.

When I returned from Italy, I decided that I wanted to learn how to take performance to the next level by getting a personal training certification. I felt that the certification would divulge some amazing secrets as to how to achieve better performance.

In 2004, I actually did two different training certifications (SMART and ISSA). I revamped my training and diet to reflect what I learned.

I recently reviewed one of my note-taking sessions and it read, (underlined) "every time that you open your mouth to eat, you should be putting protein in." So that's what I did. I ate lots of nuts and cottage cheese, fish, whey protein, casein protein, protein bars, soy protein: carbs were the enemy!

I looked really muscular (though I had a little belly) and thought, "this will be my best season ever!"

But a funny thing happened. I kept pulling muscles all of the time. My back was tight. I was always tired. Plus, I found that my performance in games wasn't actually any better.

I was like, "What gives?"

The problem, in retrospect, was that I became a bodybuilder. I was not doing functional training that was appropriate for my sport. Not only that, but without carbohydrates, athletes really have inadequate fuel for workouts and competitions. I learned how wasteful inappropriate training is several years later, after much research and an amazing trip where I shadowed the Director of Sports Performance (Brandon Marcello) at Stanford University in California.

That is why I became obsessed with proper training and recovery methods.

I unfortunately learned much of this information after I had already stopped my pitching career to focus more on my developing business, but *you* can now benefit from all of my research. Plus, even without the huge advantage that this information affords, I continued to have success. Until, seemingly out of nowhere, I couldn't find the strike zone. Just as a note to my readers, I was always a little wild, but that was part of my movement and effectiveness. This was different. I was definitely in my head in a way that I hated. I didn't know where to put my focus and I was actually nervous. I was playing on a team of such great athletes and I didn't want to let them down. I hated what I was feeling and knew I had to do something about it. I had gone for a few hypnosis sessions when I was younger and remembered that being very helpful, so I decided to give it a try for sports performance.

It was like a small miracle.

That is why I became certified as a hypnotist. Truthfully, most athletes go through something similar to what I experienced, and it can be debilitating. I wanted to be able to help them.

That is why I became obsessed with addressing the mental aspect of performance.

The last year that I pitched competitively, I was really not feeling well in general. I had a very good season overall, but I had constant congestion, aching joints, dizziness, headaches and weight loss. Things continued to digress after my last competitive season was over. In a short period of time, I had torn my posterior tibial tendon, herniated a disc in my back, experienced frequent muscle spasms, breathing issues, and pervasive fatigue. I then started getting stomach pains that seemed to get worse all of the time. Blood-work and other tests did seem to reveal something was wrong, but no one could give me a definitive answer as to what it was or what I could do to help matters.

Friends and family kept telling me that feeling unwell all the time was a result of being so active. Plus, I was in my late twenties. It gets harder as you get older, they said. They felt that my body needed time to rest.

I never believed a word of that.

I know what fatigue and burnout feel like. I knew that something wasn't right, and kept going for tests and exams until a few doctors speculated that I probably had the beginning of an autoimmune condition.

I was pretty devastated. There isn't a whole lot that anyone can do about an autoimmune condition, right?

Just as I was resigning myself to living with the way I felt, which seemed pretty miserable, something magical happened.

I followed my curiosity.

I love adventure and seeking out new places and things. My husband and I had wanted to go to Costa Rica for a long time, and finally decided to do a tour via bus. We met a lot of interesting people and had an amazing time. Three people in particular really stood out, though. They were sweet, interesting, highly intelligent and vegans. The vegan part understandably generated a lot of questions, especially since we all ate together. The servers typically had to make some modifications for our new friends.

For those of you getting ready to run screaming at the use of the word "vegan," don't be afraid. This book focuses specifically on how eating this way (or even mostly this way) will help you to become more alkaline, healthy, and recover faster. Though animal treatment and environmental issues are important, they will not be addressed in this book.

Many people are not really sure what being "vegan" really means. I had known a little more about veganism than the rest of the group in Costa Rica since I had been a pescatarian (a vegetarian who also eats fish) for about 3 years at that point. I thought veganism seemed like something that would be nearly impossible to sustain on a daily basis, since it avoids all animal products entirely (meaning no dairy, eggs, or fish). My macho personal training certification was whispering in my ear, "there is no way they are getting enough protein." It was even whispering something along the lines of "because they are vegan, they must be weak." It is embarrassing to say that now, but it was true at the time.

But I was proven completely wrong.

While horseback riding, they were trotting happily along in the front while I was shivering and plodding away in the back. They had seemingly endless energy during hikes and still had enough left at night to stay up and party with my husband and the group tour guide (I was already in bed at that time).

I was forced to re-evaluate some admittedly very biased thinking. Maybe my magical personal training certification had been wrong about diet?

Gasp!

Scandal!

I was now very curious about what it would be like to eat vegan. So when I got home, I committed to trying it for two weeks.

So if you are thinking you are about to read something about how it was all sunshine, rainbows, and unicorns the second I stopped eating eggs, fish, and dairy, sorry to disappoint. It was not easy at all at first. I loved eating eggs every morning, and I went completely cold turkey. I also had what I would classify as a mild addiction to sushi and cheese, and avoiding all of that was really tough to come to terms with. I initially didn't really understand the idea that most of my nutrition should have been coming from vegetables. I was still so focused on protein, carbs and fat, and it took a while to change that mindset.

Regardless, after the two weeks, I started to feel less tired and achy. I was more clear-headed. I had more energy.

I was kind of shocked. How was this happening without the copious amounts of protein that are supposedly necessary for athletes? Later, I learned exactly why this was the case, but it was very confusing at the time. In fact, later we will discuss how too much protein can actually be tough on your digestion and negatively affect performance.

After about three weeks of eating a vegan diet, I gave in to the siren call of sushi. I didn't get violently ill or anything like that. I just felt kind of foggy and grumpy the whole day. I wasn't as focused and didn't feel all that great energy. That cemented it. I haven't had any animal products at all since that day.

So I decided to keep at the whole vegan thing, despite the fact that my parents were now beside themselves. While out to dinner at a fancy restaurant, mom informed the waiter, "well, Jules has gone *vegan* (pronounce "vegan" with the same sort of bitter quality you would use for the words "serial killer")." It can admittedly be challenging at times.

But I feel amazing every day.

I have only had 3 colds over the span of 4 years. I don't usually need an alarm to wake up in the morning. I am really rarely sore.

So if you are reading this right now and thinking, "There is no way in hell that I am becoming a vegan!" fear not, my friend. I do recommend going entirely plant-based if you can, but I also realize that can be very difficult for some people. Even if you don't cut out animal products entirely, eating a lot less of them and focusing on lots of green vegetables and fruits will still yield great benefits.

Plus, even if you are a die-hard meat-eater, you will still reap the benefits of this book.

After several months of being vegan and feeling great all of the time, I knew that my time in sports was not yet done. Pitching, however, was very difficult because of team practices and game schedules. I couldn't commit to these the way I wanted to while simultaneously running a business. Running, on the other hand, was quite easy. I could do it at any time of day or night and I didn't need anyone else to practice with. So I started running some local races and was pleasantly surprised to find that I always placed really well for my age bracket.

Most importantly, I felt great and was never sore afterwards.

I ran my first half-marathon with minimal training (not something I would really advise, but I know about recovery, so I managed).

Then I decided that I really needed to put my diet, recovery and athletic capabilities to the ultimate test.

I decided to join CrossFit.

Now, I made sure that I joined a very reputable Crossfit where form was prioritized over everything (remember I am obsessed with good form and movement), but it is still important to be careful. Crossfit generally emphasizes going up in weight constantly and that isn't always smart. Just because you can do it for one or two reps, doesn't mean you should.

Even after On-ramp (the program they do at the beginning to make sure that you know all of the moves), where most people are dying sore, I felt fine. I actually felt even more energized and excited for our daily competitions.

Just to be straight, though, I am not very good at CrossFit. Just like pitching, I realize I am slow to learn the new movements and certainly haven't perfected them. I definitely get that look from the coaches quite often that reads, "it's okay, we know you are a little slow to catch on." I will keep plugging away, though, and since I can train harder and recover faster, I will be decent at it eventually.

Just today I did my very first workout without subs (easier substitutions) and I feel like I just conquered the world.

So, this is why I became obsessed with nutrient density and nutrition.

It changed everything about how I feel, perform and act. It even has promoted a sense of well-being in me that is pretty hard to shake.

Lucky you: you are about to discover the most amazing secrets to fluid movements, training, recovery, nutrition and the mental aspect of the game. It took me nearly 15 years to compile all of this information. It will change your performance. It will change your mindset. It will allow you to do things that you never thought you could do.

3

2

1

Go!

CHAPTER TWO:
PERFORMANCE MISTAKES TO AVOID

You take your sport very seriously. You have a coach who works with you on your mechanics. You do weight training and cross-training. You belong to a travel organization that plays year round. You might even try to eat pretty well.

So why aren't you going out and kicking ass every day?

You should be the best at your sport. You don't want to feel run-down and worn out.

Unfortunately, there are many common mistakes that people make that can destroy the ability to perform at optimal levels.

Granted, if you don't have good coordination or the right build for your sport, you probably won't reach Olympic-level skill no matter what you do.

On the other side of that, there are a lot of little things that you can change that can make you achieve your true potential. It's a terrible feeling to think that you have hit a wall either with training or with skill development.

I personally don't think anyone should hit a wall at any age.

Unless, of course, you are breaking world records, in which case, that is a pretty good wall to stop at. You can just enjoy the beautiful view at that particular wall.

So below are a few things that can contribute to inflammation, fatigue, and sub-par performance. We will discuss these items in more detail throughout the book, but even one or two of these little buggers can bring your progress to a grinding halt:

Overtraining: Yes, there is such a thing! If you don't schedule rest and recovery time, your body will schedule it for you: generally in the form of an injury or illness. Soft tissue does need time to repair, even with the best recovery system. If you follow the guidelines laid out for you in this book, you will recover in less time, but you still need to use good judgment, especially if you are an asymmetrical athlete (like a pitcher or tennis player). Asymmetrical athletes mostly use only one side of their body and therefore tend to tax a few muscle groups all the time. This often leads to the muscles developing in a way that is not very balanced. There are several signs and symptoms indicating that rest might be the best option for your development. We will discuss these in Chapter Seven. Additionally, know that your body doesn't actually build muscle while in the gym. "*What?!,*" you say. I know it sounds crazy, but it is a fact. Working out creates tiny tears in the muscle and building muscle is your body's response to repair damaged tissue. The thing is, if you just keep damaging the muscles over and over again, your body has no time to repair the damaged tissue. That means you are in a constant state of breaking down, with no opportunity to build.

Lack of "Deep Practice": Maybe you train just the right amount, but you are still not making progress. You are working on your skills every other day and do cross-training on off-days. You are wondering why all of your practice doesn't seem to be getting you anywhere. Well, there's practice and then there's *deep practice*. I work with athletes every day and everyone wants a formula for success that goes something like this:

100 of drill y x 6 days a week = guaranteed success

The truth is, a formula like that will never be accurate, because some athletes will perform those repetitions while they are talking to their friends or thinking about what they are going to wear the next day. Other athletes will perform those repetitions by breaking them down, examining where they were strong versus where they were weak, and literally improving on each repetition. Some athletes will imagine game situations while they practice and develop different scenarios and obstacles to overcome. Other athletes will do practice just to "get through it." You cannot compare the effectiveness of these forms of practice. To be successful, you must have a good understanding of working without distraction and with determination. Each practice should be designed to overcome at least one thing that you have been struggling with. Team practice doesn't count! You are simply not getting enough repetitions to better yourself at a team practice. Team practice is generally more focused on how you interact with your teammates during plays and how you communicate with them in different situations. Working on the *skills* that will make you great is a task that falls on you alone. Practice with intention, a critical perspective, and awareness of your movements.

Improper Warm Up: Is it bad that I want to gag every time I watch a team lap around the field and then static stretch for twenty minutes while they chat with their friends about pretty much everything but the upcoming practice/game? Everyone needs to warm up. Muscles are like wax. If you are cold and try to be explosive with them, they will get injured. If you try to stretch them when they are not warm, they will also get injured. But too many athletes just do a run-of-the-mill warm up without taking the needs of their specific sport into question. Your pre-workout movements should specifically address anything that is already uncomfortable from previous workouts and should specifically prep you for the workout you are about to do. You need a focused, dynamic warm-up where every motion you make is done with intention and done to help you in your sport. This should include (at the very least): warming the muscles, using the foam roller, and going through different planes of motion (just like in competition).

Improper Recovery Techniques: This is where most athletes tend to fail. I am going to include bad diet under "improper recovery," since bad diet can limit recovery to a very large extent. We will discuss diet in depth in later chapters, but there are many other factors that affect recovery. Cooling down after intense activity should be where your recovery process starts. This allows your body to readjust to being inactive. Plus, your muscles will generally be very tight after a hard workout, so you should do some static stretching after cooling down (or as part of a cool down). This is especially important if you are traveling and need to sit on a bus or a van for a long period after activity. Muscles that are already tight will get really stiff if you haven't cooled down or stretched and then proceed to sit for long periods of time. Athletes who fail to ice overtaxed muscles also tend to experience more inflammation, deteriorating performance, and oftentimes injury. Hearing "I didn't ice it because it never hurt before" is like nails on a blackboard to me. Let's just put a big "duh" sticker on that one since you should be icing anything that is getting the crap knocked out of it over and over again. Just don't ice for over twenty minutes since that limits the effectiveness of icing and risks freezing the tissue. Pulsing (hot and cold) has also become popular, and even ice baths can be used, depending on your specific needs. Just be cautious with ice baths, particularly if you don't have good circulation. Finally, getting enough sleep is a huge part of the recovery process. Your body repairs and rebuilds while you sleep. Lack of sleep can lead to compromised focus, coordination, and mechanics. The sleep-deprived also have an increased risk of injury.

Bad Mechanics: If you practice a lot but poorly, it still won't help you improve. Many athletes come in to see me for the first time complaining that they work hard and practice all the time but don't see any improvement. We adjust the movements of the body and we have some *Harry Potter* kind of magic. I have had some athletes improve pitch speed by as much as 4-5 mph in a week. It is therefore essential to find a coach specific to your sport that really knows what he or she is doing. The problem I see very often is that athletes will learn from someone who has a huge list of accomplishments in a specific sport, but no background in personal training, biomechanics, physics, or anything that would give them greater awareness about how the body is supposed to move to increase efficiency and avoid injury. Now, such a background isn't absolutely necessary, but when you are shopping around for a coach, at the very least consider their track record. Does this particular coach have athletes who have achieved a very high level of success? What about the rate of injury? Does the coach you're looking at typically have a lot of girls out on injury? If so, why are you even considering using her? Also, does the coach you are thinking of using subscribe to a specific set of ideals no matter what or does she take differences in anatomy into account? These are very important things to consider. Great athletes can make great coaches, but they don't always. "Gifted" athletes haven't always had to struggle through lots of failure and difficulty to achieve success, so they don't always understand how to correct problems when they come face-to-face with them. It is best to choose someone who is knowledgeable, experienced, patient, and has a good rapport with you.

Clueless about Hydration: Your low energy levels can simply have to do with being mildly dehydrated. This is not all that uncommon. Here are some sneaky things that might be dehydrating you: drinking a lot of caffeine/diuretics, drinking only when you are thirsty, not ever having electrolytes.

You Think You are Eating Well, but You are Not: So you skipped breakfast, had lunch at 10:30 am, had a game at 4:00 and didn't eat again until after 7. Even if you ate a diet composed of the best types of foods, your performance would still suffer because your nutrient timing sucks. *What* you eat is really important, but also *when* you eat. If you are clueless on both ends, you simply cannot perform optimally. Ask yourself, "do I really know what my body needs to fuel an intense workout?"

Too Much Stress/ or Not Enough: As my mentor wrote in his book *Swag 101*, "I always run faster when a dog is chasing me." This means that when the competition is heavy and intense, he will perform his best. On the other hand, you might be suffering from too much stress. Although my coaching method is mostly patient with a lot of different ways to describe things, I typically thrive as an athlete when someone is screaming at me. I can't really explain that, but it is just the way it is. It gets me mad; it motivates me. Some athletes are completely the opposite and can't be talked at with even a stern voice. You have to decide what level of stress you operate best at. For me, it is against the big competition with the stakes high. For other athletes, that pressure is too much. Find your balance through experimentation.

There's too much going on in your head: Most high-level athletes are going to have to deal with some inner demons at one point or another. As a hypnotist, I find the best way to really solve this problem in a long-lasting way is to find out the EXACT reason why the difficulty started in the first place. Trace your mental discomfort back to the first time it ever happened. Consider the events that were occurring in your life at the time. Were your parents in the middle of a divorce? Did a close friend or coach die? Did you recently move? Most people think that these variables have very little to do with athletic performance, but anything that weighs heavily on your mind can also affect your body. If you can't work it out yourself, seek help. There are so many people out there who can help you. You don't have to suffer alone.

CHAPTER THREE:
SIZE REALLY DOESN'T MATTER (MEET THE MICRONUTRIENTS)

"Bottom line: If you're trying to keep sick days at bay, stick to nutrient dense foods. . –Roshini Rajapaksa, MD [1]

Although most athletes are familiar with macronutrients (fat, protein, and carbs), they usually know very little about micronutrients. What are micronutrients? They are vitamins, minerals and antioxidants. So why are these little guys so important? They are the raw materials that your body uses to send nerve signals, create chemical messages, produce muscle, and perform many other tasks.[2] Our bodies do not produce enough of these nutrients on their own. It is therefore essential that we take these nutrients in via food to keep the chemical processes running smoothly, recover faster from tough workouts, and keep the immune system functioning at its best. Though you might feel a little run down if you don't have enough protein on board, not having enough vitamin C can cause scurvy (yes, like a pirate). Severe B12 deficiency can cause pernicious anemia (which is irreversible). There are many more examples, but this is why micronutrients are the unsung heroes of the nutritional world, particularly for athletes.

---

[1] Rajapaksa, Roshini. (2014, April 20). "Our Doc Will See you Now." *Health.* 72.

[2] http://www.helpguide.org/harvard/vitamins_and_minerals.htm

In fact, many people who have ongoing issues with food cravings, moodiness, or inconsistent performance might be showing signs of what is referred to as a "subclinical nutrient deficiency." This is a term used to describe a shortage of one or more micronutrients in your body. This shortage is enough to affect health and/or mood, but not quite enough to show typical deficiency symptoms that might be recognized by your health care provider. This can be a very involved and complicated topic and this chapter took me *forever* to write. So you better use it! I will give you basic information about micronutrients followed by summaries about each, what they do in the body, and signs of deficiency. If you don't want to read the whole chapter, you can just use it as a "mini reference book" on micronutrients. If you are confused or overwhelmed after reading it, that would be a good time to have me come and speak for your organization.

Right now you are probably thinking, "but I take a multivitamin. I should have all of the vitamins and minerals I need." You might be surprised. We tend to get less than 2/3 of the magnesium we need.[3] If you are an athlete, this is especially troublesome, since magnesium is a mineral that is incredibly important for recovery and muscle contractions. About 75% of us don't meet the Recommended Daily Allowance for Folate or Calcium.[4] Plus, Vitamin D deficiency seems to be a growing epidemic.

So what gives?

We don't generally get enough micronutrients because the American diet is so filled with over-processed and genetically modified foods. If you head down the cereal, bread or snack aisle, you are going to find a veritable wasteland of processed foods. Anything that you buy at a fast food chain is also guaranteed to be processed to an absurd degree and probably also genetically modified. How else do you know if something is processed? It usually has about a million ingredients (many of which you can't

---

[3] Ansel, Karen. (2014 May). Eating Wisely. *Yoga Journal.* Issue 264. 38.
[4] United States Department of Agriculture, 2009

pronounce) and so many preservatives that it won't expire until sometime after you do. When in doubt, follow the motto of one of my favorite snack companies: "if it doesn't go bad, it's not good for you."

Processing food is so bad because it strips foods of their vitamins and minerals, leaving a hollow shell of nutrition. Plus, lots of sugar and fillers are usually added to make the "food product" palatable. All of the preservatives added to these foods generally pass FDA screenings through what amounts to an honor system.[5] That is a terrifying fact when you consider how much money is at stake when a company realizes that they can make a "food product" that can last through an apocalypse. The ingredients in some of these things are so scary that Satan himself probably wouldn't touch them, even if it were the end of the world. These preservatives have been implicated in everything from ADHD to various health conditions, and the research is relatively limited on their long-term affects.

Ready to give up processed foods, yet?

NO?

I understand: they are convenient. Plus, you might pick up a box of say, Cinnamon Toast Crunch, read the label, and be pleasantly surprised to discover that there are somehow magically some vitamins in there. Not so fast. Synthetic vitamins are sometimes sprayed onto foods after all the nutrients have been processed out, but it is not quite the same as getting the real thing.

---

[5] Warner, Melanie. (2013). *Pandora's Lunchbox.* New York: Scribner.

Over the last several years, "nutritionism" has emerged. In "nutritionism" (or substitute "being an idiot," if you want to be real) certain nutrients get made into rock stars. We claim that these are the most important ones (really!) and then they appear in everything from pill form to synthetic ingredients in "food products." The idea that only a few nutrients are making your entire amazing biological system work at its best is pure nonsense.

The truth is, vitamins and minerals work harmoniously in real food (read: "fruits and vegetables"), but may not do so when taken as an isolated supplement that was created in a laboratory. Additionally, taking too much of one supplement can make it difficult for the other micronutrients to be absorbed properly. For example, too much manganese can make iron deficiency worse.[6] On the other side of that, let's look at nature's perfection in the form of an orange. When you eat an orange, you are not just eating isolated (or synthetic!) vitamin C, you are also eating potassium, magnesium, calcium and iron[7]! These nutrients work together in your body to conduct chemical processes and help speed up healing, among other things. As another example, magnesium helps calcium and potassium ions to travel across cell membranes, something that is very important for conducting nerve impulses and muscle contractions.[8] In other words, if you are just taking a calcium supplement, you are getting some of that supplement in your body, but you might not be getting it to where it needs to go to be effective without the help of the other micronutrients. Plus, if the calcium is not sourced properly, one reason why I am obsessive about only using certain brands, you may actually be causing more harm than good by taking supplements.

One of the theorized reasons why the current population cannot seem to get enough Vitamin D is the fact that, even if you take a huge dose of synthetic Vitamin D in isolation, you are probably not getting the *other*

---

[6] http://www.helpguide.org/harvard/vitamins_and_minerals.htm
[7] http://www.health-alternatives.com/fruit-nutrition-chart.html
[8] http://ods.od.nih.gov/factsheets/Magnesium-HealthProfessional/

micronutrients that will complement it and help your body absorb it (like Vitamin K).[9] This would be one reason why a person could take a massive amount of Vitamin D and still show a deficiency (though there could be other reasons as well).

These are some of the many reasons why it is better to get your nutrients from food sources. It is hard to *eat* too much of a particular micronutrient, but you can definitely get too much in pill or supplement form.

Another reason why eating your vitamins and minerals is superior to taking them in pill form is the fact that synthetic vitamins are missing the mineral activators, co-factors, enzymes and co-vitamin helpers that occur in nature.[10] Additionally, if the vitamins you are taking in pill form are produced cheaply, they are likely composed of more suspect chemicals and fillers. They might even contain genetically modified ingredients. So let's get to know some micronutrients and some good ways to eat them (not swallow them in a pill).

First of all, what is the difference between vitamins and minerals? Vitamins can be broken down by heat, air, or acid, but minerals keep their chemical structure.[11]

This is important because it means that minerals in food don't degrade with transport, storage, cooking and exposure to elements the same way that vitamins do. This is one of the many reasons why eating local and organic is important: if kale has to travel in a truck for a week and then sit in a warehouse before you consume it, you are losing vital nutrients.

---

[9] Precision Nutrition: http://www.precisionnutrition.com/stop-vitamin-d
[10] http://energyfanatics.com/2008/10/19/how-to-natural-synthetic-vitamins/
[11] http://www.helpguide.org/harvard/vitamins_and_minerals.htm

Organic foods have also been shown to be higher in vitamins and minerals then conventionally grown produce.

So now you know that you aren't getting anything good out of synthetic foods, but you are probably wondering about all of the amazing vitamins and minerals out there, what they do, and how you can eat them. If, while reading the rest of this chapter, you find that you are questioning your will to live, how do you think I felt writing it? All kidding aside, though, if these things don't interest you, feel free to skip ahead to the next chapter. I wouldn't, though, since this is some really important stuff and I have tried to make it as digestible as possible (okay, bad pun). Even if you skip it now, however, use it in the future to determine what you might be lacking (or potentially getting too much of). Here are some vitamins, how they are broken down, and how to consume them:

WATER SOLUBLE VITAMINS

Water-soluble vitamins go into your bloodstream while food is broken down during digestion. Since the body is mostly made of water, these vitamins usually circulate easily in the body.[12] Water-soluble vitamins include B vitamins and vitamin C.

B Vitamins

What do B Vitamins Do?

All B vitamins are used to help the body make food into the fuel that produces energy. They help the body to break down fats and protein, and help the nervous system to function properly.[13] There are several different types of B vitamins:

---

[12] http://www.helpguide.org/harvard/vitamins_and_minerals.htm
[13] http://umm.edu/health/medical/altmed/supplement/vitamin-h-biotin

The Details on B7

-B7 occurs naturally in foods, while "biotin" is produced synthetically (19).

-You need B7 to properly use the carbs, fats and amino acids[14] that you eat.

-Vegetarians absorb B7 better than omnivores because of the way gut bacteria changes on a vegetarian diet[15].

-Alcohol gets in the way of using and absorbing B7.

-B7 has been used for the treatment of skin conditions and diabetes.

Signs of B7 deficiency

-Muscle pain, low energy, dry skin[16] brittle hair and nails (13).

Food sources of B7

-Brown rice, whole grains, legumes, peanuts, cauliflower, mushrooms, soybeans, nuts and nut butters, and bananas (13).

The Details on B9

-Folate (vitamin b9) occurs naturally in foods, while "folic acid" is produced synthetically and found in many industrialized foods.[17]

-Folate plays a huge role in creating neurotransmitters and DNA (15).

-It is vital for formation of red blood cells.

[14] umm.edu

[15] Kirschmann, J. D. 7 Nutrition Search, Inc. (2007). *Nutrition Almanac (Sixth Edition)*. USA: McGraw-Hill.

[16] Kirschmann, J. D. 7 Nutrition Search, Inc. (2007). *Nutrition Almanac (Sixth Edition)*. USA: McGraw-Hill.

[17] http://www.globalhealingcenter.com/natural-health/folic-acid-foods/

-It is involved in forming myelin, which is important for brain function. Myelin is built along a specific pathway when you are learning a new skill or athletic movement. Once myelin is built along the correct pathway, athletic movements are made smoother, better, and more familiar. They also can be done faster. For those of you who haven't, read *The Talent Code* yet, it is a must-read for a wonderful explanation of how practice leads to myelin formation in the body.

-Folate is an important part of mental and emotional health (15).

-It can play a role in preventing cardiovascular disease.

-It is very important for pregnant women since it mostly affects cells that are rapidly dividing.

Signs of B9 deficiency

-Feeling depressed and irritable, forgetting things, having trouble with digestion, and stomach upset (15).

Food sources of B9

- Folate is easily destroyed by exposure to light or heat. That means that cooking the fruits and vegetables listed below will diminish their folate content (lentils and beans must be cooked or sprouted before they are eaten, however): green leafy plants (spinach, kale, etc.), brown rice, citrus fruits, asparagus, broccoli, beans, lentils, avocado, Brussels Sprouts, nuts, seeds, cauliflower, beets, celery, carrots, squash, wheat grass, chlorella, flaxseed, and kelp.[18]

---

[18] http://www.globalhealingcenter.com/natural-health/folic-acid-foods/

The Details on B3

-Vitamin B3 is found naturally in foods and "Niacin" is produced synthetically. [19]

-B3 is pretty stable because it is resistant to heat, light, and air.

-It is made in the body from protein, particularly tryptophan.

-It helps to break down and use proteins, fats and carbs.

-It is needed to keep the nervous system functioning at its best. It helps to form and maintain healthy skin, tongue and digestive system tissues.

-It is necessary to synthesize sex hormones.

-It supports detoxification (20).

-It is used in the treatment of joint disease (20).

-It has calming effects and can contribute to mental well-being, better sleep and treatment of depression. (20)

-You will need more of this when you are ill, have sustained an injury or are going through a period of growth.

-Eating too much starch and sugar will reduce the body's supply of B3.

Signs of B3 deficiency

-Problems with the skin, upset stomach, fatigue, muscle weakness, indigestion, and sometimes anxiety disorders. Headaches, insomnia, and irritability are also signs of deficiency (20).

---

[19] http://energyfanatics.com/2008/10/19/how-to-natural-synthetic-vitamins/)

Food sources of B3

-Whole grains (not corn), legumes, peanuts, mushrooms, peas, sunflower seeds, chia seeds, sesame seeds, figs, bananas, wheatgrass and avocados (20). Foods high in tryptophan yield B3.

The Details on B5

-Vitamin B5 is found naturally in foods and "pantothenic acid" is the synthetic form of B5.

-It is found in *all* living cells.

-In the body, B5 takes the form of a coenzyme that is a vital part of Krebs cycle energy production.[20] The Krebs cycle is a part of how the body uses oxygen to make food separate into nutrients to create energy. Athletes and people who exercise regularly are engaging in this cycle very frequently.

-Evidence shows a connection between levels of B5 in the body and strong performance of the outer portion of the adrenal glands (adrenal cortex). The adrenal cortex puts out hormones that effect metabolism and chemicals in the blood. Specifically, the adrenal cortex secretes cortisol, corticosterone, aldosterone hormone, and androgenic steroids. Cortisol, along with adrenaline, is responsible for that fight or flight edge in in competition. Cortisol also affects how we use fats, protein and carbs. Corticosterone affects inflammation in the body and immune function. The aldosterone hormone limits the amount of sodium you release in urine. This is important for athletes since we need to maintain good levels of electrolytes and good blood volume and pressure. Androgenic steroids are essentially your body's own anabolic steroids.[21]

---

[20] Kirschmann, J. D. 7 Nutrition Search, Inc. (2007). *Nutrition Almanac (Sixth Edition)*. USA: McGraw-Hill.

[21] http://umm.edu/programs/diabetes/health/endocrinology-health-guide/adrenal-glands

-Since B5 can have such positive affect on the adrenal glands, it can improve the body's ability to deal with stressful conditions.

-B5 has a reputation for improving athletic ability (20).

-B5 helps build antibodies for fighting infection.

-It is involved in the synthesis of many other vitamins.

Signs of B5 deficiency

-B5 deficiency is typically only an issue if the flora inside of the intestine is not healthy and therefore can't synthesize B5. Most people get enough in their diet. If deficiency does occur, signs are reduced immunity to infections, hypoglycemia, sensitivity to insulin, insomnia, fatigue, and depression (20).

Food sources of B5

Peanuts, pecans, oatmeal, shiitake mushrooms, avocado, sweet potato, lentils, peas, and broccoli.

The Details on B2

-B2 is found naturally in foods while "riboflavin" is the synthetic form of B2.

-B2 plays a huge role in energy production. It is stored in the muscles and used in times of physical exertion, so it is extremely important for anyone who exercises (20).

-B2 works inside the cell and also protects the cell from damage (20).

-It helps to maintain appropriate levels of powerful antioxidants.

-It helps the body to process and use several other nutrients.

-It protects against free-radical damage that follows exercise. B2 is associated with improved athletic performance (19).

-It is important for good skin, nails, and hair.

Signs of B2 Deficiency

Inadequate levels of B2 can result in anemia.

Food sources of B2

Dark leafy greens, almonds, soybeans, spinach, tempeh, asparagus, and crimini mushrooms.

The Details on B1

-B1 occurs naturally in foods while "thiamin hydrochloride" and "thiamin mononitrate" are synthetic forms of B1.

-B1 has a huge role in the process of converting carbohydrates, proteins, and fats into energy (20).

-It is important for good nervous system functioning.

-B1 helps to create a strong immune system.

-B1 is associated with a better ability to learn.

-It helps to maintain heart and red blood cells.

-It helps to regulate appetite by helping with the digestion and use of food (20).

-It is needed in order to create hydrochloric acid, which helps digestion (20).

Signs of B1 Deficiency

Beriberi, weight loss, gastrointestinal issues, weakness, high blood pressure, heart issues, nausea, headaches, and weight loss.

Food Sources of B1

Legumes, collard greens, unprocessed rice, wheatgrass, and blackstrap molasses.[22]

The Details on B6

- Vitamin B6 occurs naturally in foods while "pyridoxine hydrochloride" is the synthetic version of B6.

-It is used to convert one amino acid into another.

-It has a huge role in the creation of protein compounds. These would include, but not be limited to, immune system cells, hormones, brain chemicals, and DNA.

-It plays a role in creating hormone-like substances that affect body processes like muscle contractions.

-It is required for the correct functioning of more than sixty enzymes (20).

-It is a part of the energy cycle because it sets off the release of glycogen from the liver and muscles.

-B6 is extremely important for athletes and anyone who exercises regularly since B6 helps to maintain the balance of sodium and potassium in the

---

[22] http://energyfanatics.com/2008/10/19/how-to-natural-synthetic-vitamins/

body: you know these two minerals as electrolytes. Electrolytes are essential for regulation of body fluids. You need them in order for your nervous and musculoskeletal systems to function at their best (20).

-It helps regulate estrogen and progesterone and therefore helps PMS (20)

Signs of B6 Deficiency

Depression, glucose intolerance, bad nerve function, skin problems, trouble learning, irritability, weakness, and nervousness (20).

Food sources of B6

The most stable form of this nutrient is found almost completely in plant foods: bananas, sunflower seeds, walnuts, spinach, and sweet potatoes.

The Details on B12

- Vitamin B12 occurs naturally in foods while "streptomycin fermentation" and "cyanocobalamin" are synthetic forms of B12.

-Remember the myelin sheath that is so important for creating consistent athletic skills? B12 is necessary for creating the myelin sheath that goes around nerve cells. It speeds up the movement of signals along those nerve cells (20). For more information on myelin, read *The Talent Code.*

-B12 plays a role in normal functioning of nerve tissue.

-B12 affects the metabolism of protein, fat, and carbohydrate (19).

-B12 helps form normal red blood cells.

-B12 helps iron to function better in the body.

-B12 helps promote absorption of other vitamins.

-It helps to improve energy levels (20), particularly in cases of chronic fatigue.

-It can stimulate metabolism (20).

-It can help you recover faster from bacterial and viral infections.

Signs of B12 Deficiency

Your body does store some B12, so a deficiency can sometimes take years to show up. However, when it does show up, it can degrade into pernicious anemia. This creates an environment in which the body does not have enough healthy red blood cells, which is dangerous for many reasons. Nerve damage and neurological problems can also result. Deficiencies also generally affect the brain and nervous system, so I advise you to be ABSOLUTELY CERTAIN that you are getting enough of this in your diet. Other signs of deficiency include sore and weak arms and legs, less reflex response, and memory loss (20). A B12 deficiency can actually mimic Alzheimer's and can also be a source of depression.

Food sources of B12

Nutritional yeast, kombucha, and bee pollen. Vitamin B12 is actually a bacteria, so fermented foods do contain small amounts. Vegetarians and vegans should consider a well-sourced supplement. I like the Innate Brand "B-Complex". Innate sources its vitamins from food, so it is one of the only brands I trust in the supplement industry.

I also like their "B-complex" since it is important to include all of the B Vitamins in your diet. Constantly taking in one type of B vitamin more than another (for example, always taking B12 but not getting enough of the other B vitamins) can make you lose the other B vitamins through urine (20).

The Details on C

- Vitamin C occurs naturally in foods while "ascorbic acid," "calcium ascorbate," and "ester C" are synthetic forms.

-Vitamin C is very unstable and sensitive to light, heat and air. You will therefore get more Vitamin C from raw, fresh fruits and vegetables than you will from cooked fruits and vegetables. Produce that has been sitting in a warehouse for a long time will contain lower levels of Vitamin C.

-Vitamin C creates collagen: a protein that is essential for forming connective tissue, tendons, and cartilage (20).

-Vitamin C helps form connective tissue in scars and so it is important for speeding the healing of wounds and/or burns.

-Vitamin C is important for the development of healthy gums.

-Vitamin C helps to stop you from bruising easily.

-Vitamin C is also an antioxidant.

-It fights bacterial infections and the common cold.

-Vitamin C prevents hemorrhaging (20).

-Vitamin C has an important role in the body's absorption of other minerals. It also helps turn tryptophan into serotonin (20)

-We have to eat vitamin C many times a day because it is out of the body in 3-4 hours (20).

-We need more Vitamin C during times of stress, infection, injury, and fatigue.

-Vitamin C helps the fluid that lubricates the joints to thin, allowing freer movement (20).

Signs of Vitamin C Deficiency

Scurvy is a result of not enough vitamin C. Early signs include fatigue, weakness, swollen arms and legs, and difficulty breathing. Other signs of deficiency include bad gums, wounds that take a long time to heal, easy bruising, constant infections, swollen and tender joints, and muscle cramps.

Food sources of Vitamin C

Citrus fruits, sweet red peppers, kale (dark leafy greens), broccoli, cauliflower, Brussels sprouts, guava, persimmons, strawberries, papaya, Camu camu and acerola cherries.

FAT SOLUBLE VITAMINS

Fat-soluble vitamins don't go directly to the bloodstream after they are digested. They actually go through the lymph vessels before going into bloodstream (11) and extra is stored in liver and fat tissues. When your body runs low, your tissues release more. Because they are stored in the body, it is possible for toxic build up to occur if you take too many supplements (11).

The Details on A

- Vitamin A occurs naturally in foods while "retinol acetate" and "retinol palmitate" are synthetic forms.

-It protects vision.

-It aids in bone formation and teeth formation.

-It helps with growth and repair of body tissues where epithelial cells (cells that line cavities and surfaces of different structures in the body) are involved.

-It is good for the skin.

-Vitamin A fights against the effects of harmful particles that might be exposed to the nose, sinuses, eyelids, mouth, throat, stomach, digestive tract, and lungs. In this way, it helps to stop these tissues from getting infected (20).

-If you engage in strenuous physical activity around the same time that you consume foods rich in Vitamin A, you might not absorb it as well as you would under other circumstances (20).

-It has been used to treat migraines (20).

-In the form of beta carotene (found in carrots), it is also an antioxidant and therefore has a role as an anti-carcinogen (20).

Signs of Vitamin A Deficiency

Night blindness, problems with the eyes, loss of sense of smell, loss of appetite, painful joints, brittle fingernails and dull hair, and weakened immune system (20).

Food sources of Vitamin A

Carrots (since beta carotene is broken down into vitamin A), beet greens, spinach, kale, butternut squash, cantaloupe, and sweet potatoes. Beta carotene is what creates the orange color in fruits and vegetables so you can tell what foods are rich in this nutrient just by the color (21).

The Details on D

-Vitamin D occurs naturally in foods while "irradiated ergosterol" and "cholecalciferol" are the synthetic forms.

-Vitamin D is produced in the body when skin is exposed to ultraviolet light (20).

-Vitamin D has a very important role in bone formation.

-It functions like a hormone.

-It can enhance immune function.

-The body needs Vitamin D in order to absorb calcium properly (20).

-Vitamin D helps stabilize the nervous system.

-Vitamin D plays a role in normal heart action and normal blood clotting.

Signs of Vitamin D Deficiency

If you are not properly absorbing calcium, low Vitamin D levels may be to blame. Low Vitamin D levels are also responsible for rickets (and osteomalacia in adults) (20). Rickets often leads to deformities and decreased muscle tone in children while osteomalacia is a softening of the bones. Bone pain and muscle weakness can be signs of Vitamin D deficiency, but sometimes symptoms are not obvious, so it is good to get your levels checked when you have blood-work done.

Food sources of Vitamin D

Some mushrooms, including shiitake, do contain Vitamin D. The best source, however, is actually sunlight! 10-15 minutes a day, 2-3 times a week is sufficient for most people.

The Details on E

- Vitamin E occurs naturally in foods while "mixed tocopherols" and "DL-alpha tocopherol" are synthetic forms.

-Vitamin E also acts as an antioxidant.

-It makes the wall of the capillaries stronger.

-It helps to prevent red blood cells from getting destroyed.

-It provides some protection against the negative effects of environmental pollutants.

-It helps prevent the deterioration of other nutrients.

-Vitamin E is very important for energy production.

-Vitamin E makes it possible for cardiac and skeletal muscles to function with less oxygen. This can improve their endurance (20).

-Vitamin E can boost the immune system.

-It helps prevent circulatory diseases.

-It helps symptoms of PMS (20).

-It helps improve bursitis and arthritis.

Signs of Vitamin E Deficiency

Nerve damage, muscle weakness, poor coordination, and involuntary eye movement (20).

Food sources of Vitamin E

Cold pressed vegetable oils, raw seeds and nuts, soybeans, asparagus, leafy greens, and brown rice.

The Details on K

- Vitamin K occurs naturally in foods and "menadione" is the synthetic form of Vitamin K.

-It has a central role in bone formation.

-It has been called the "band-aid vitamin" since it helps so much with blood clotting (20).

-Research shows that women who are lower in Vitamin K have a higher incidence of hip fractures.

-Vitamin K plays a role in storing blood sugar in cells for later use as a source of energy.

-Vitamin K is important for normal liver function.

-It can help alleviate period cramps and heavy periods (20).

-It has been helpful in the treatment and prevention of osteoporosis (20).

Signs of Vitamin K Deficiency

Deficiencies are unusual, but can occur with people who have digestive issues and are therefore not absorbing their vitamins. Signs of deficiency include bruising easily and having noticeably ruptured capillaries.

Food sources of Vitamin K

Dark leafy greens (kale, cabbage, romaine lettuce, spinach, broccoli, green tea), green peas, asparagus, wheat grass and oats (20).

MINERALS

"I will also save you a great deal of time and trouble by condensing my advice about minerals to a very few words: eat more fruits and vegetables."

-Dr. Andrew Weil

What is the difference between a major mineral and a trace mineral?

The title of "major" or "trace" does not have anything to do with how important the mineral is for overall health and function. Both major and trace minerals are incredibly important for nearly all of the reactions occurring in the body on a daily basis. The titles of "major" and "minor" are just a way of indicating how much of them your body needs. Your body needs major minerals in relatively much higher doses than it does minor minerals.[23]

MAJOR MINERALS

Calcium

The Details

-It plays a role in bone structure.

-It aids the release of neurotransmitters (including serotonin).

-It has a role in muscle stimulation, regular heartbeat, the function of the parathyroid hormone, and the clotting of blood.

-It helps to metabolize Vitamin D (20).

-It can help with insomnia.

-It is important for nerve transmission, muscle growth, and strong muscle contractions (20).

-It calms nerves and promotes deep sleep when taken before bed (20).

---

[23] http://healthyeating.sfgate.com/difference-between-major-trace-minerals-5201.html

[24] Weil, Andrew. (2000). *Eating Well for Optimum Health*. New York. Alfred A. Knopf

-It can alleviate PMS cramps and tension.

-It can lessen muscle cramps in feet and legs (20).

-Diets very high in animal protein increase the loss of calcium in the urine.[24]

Signs of Calcium Deficiency

Calcium deficiency is actually extremely common, with most people consuming only one-third to one-half of the necessary RDA. Muscle cramps, numbness, and tingling in the arms and legs (20) are all signs of calcium deficiency. Additional signs include heart palpitations, increased cholesterol levels, slow pulse rates, insomnia, impaired growth, irritability, brittle nails, and eczema. Severe cases of calcium deficiency can result in rickets or osteoporosis.

Food sources of Calcium

Tofu (if calcium chloride is used in the processing of it), leafy green veggies, kale, collard greens, peas, oranges, almonds, sesame seeds, blackstrap molasses, sea vegetables, and sesame seeds

Chloride

The Details

-Chloride is a negatively charged ion.

-It helps regulate the balance of acid and alkali in the blood (20).

-It is one of the components of the acids used to break down food in the stomach.

-It helps keep the tendons and joints healthy.

-It helps to distribute hormones (20).

Signs of Chloride Deficiency

-Deficiencies are rare in the United States, but include hair and tooth loss, poor muscle contractions and difficulty with digestion (20).

Food sources of Chloride

Sea salt, sea vegetables, olives, lettuce, tomatoes, and celery

Magnesium

The Details

-The most magnesium in the human body is found in the bones.

-It helps convert glucose into energy.

-It helps metabolize fat.

-It plays a role in transmission of impulses in muscles.

-It helps to stabilize the amount of electricity in the cells.

-It is involved in neurotransmission (20).

-It is necessary for correct functioning of muscles.

-It helps the body to properly use other vitamins and minerals.

-It might be related to the regulation of body temperature.

-It can help cramping associated with PMS (20).

Signs of Magnesium Deficiency

Deficiency is common in the United States because of how heavily processed our foods are. People who are deficient in magnesium have an increased risk of problems with the heart (20). Magnesium deficiency is also associated with osteoporosis. Symptoms of deficiency include backaches, neck pain, tension headaches, and/or muscle cramps. Low Magnesium levels can also affect mood and sense of well-being, since magnesium affects the Central Nervous System.

Food sources of Magnesium

Whole grains, beans, seeds, nuts, fresh green vegetables, cacao, soybeans, almonds, cashews, garlic, figs, and dates

Phosphorus

The Details

-The main function of phosphorous is to form bones and teeth.

-"It plays a role in how the body uses carbs and fats. It is also needed for the body to make protein for the growth, maintenance, and repair of cells and tissues. Phosphorus also helps the body make ATP, a molecule the body uses to store energy" (20).

-It works with B vitamins and helps with:

-kidney function

-muscle contractions

-normal heartbeat

-nerve signaling[25]

---

[25] http://www.nlm.nih.gov/medlineplus/ency/article/002424.htm

Signs of Phosphorous Deficiency

Reduced appetite, anemia, muscle pain, bad bone formation (rickets), numbness and weakened immune system[26]

Food sources of Phosphorous

Phosphorous is found in almost every food. Pumpkin seeds, brazil nuts, soybeans, beans and lentils, cocoa powder, poppy seeds, sundried tomatoes, watercress, shitake mushrooms, portabella mushrooms, white mushrooms, buckwheat, and peanut butter are all good sources, but there are many others as well.[27]

Potassium

The Details

-It has a role in how nerves transmit and how muscles contract.

-Potassium helps facilitate proper enzymatic reactions (20).

-It combines with phosphorous to send oxygen to the brain.

-It works with calcium to regulate neuromuscular function.

-It is required for the synthesis of muscle protein and protein compounds in the blood.

-It helps keep skin healthy and the body alkaline (more on alkalinity later).

---

[26] http://www.healthaliciousness.com/articles/high-phosphorus-foods.php

[27] http://www.healthaliciousness.com/articles/high-phosphorus-foods.php

-Potassium and sodium help to regulate water balance in body and keep a normal heartbeat.

-It helps transfer nutrients to cells.

-You can lose it when you sweat.

-Athletes typically need more potassium than the average person.

-Almost all fruits are great sources.

-Dark, leafy greens and root vegetables are other great sources (24).

Signs of Potassium Deficiency

Muscle weakness, irritability, and rapid heartbeat are all signs of deficiency. Over the long term, low levels of potassium have been associated with fragile bones (20). Sweating from exercise on a regular basis can contribute to potassium deficiency, so athletes need to make sure they are getting enough. In athletes, muscle weakness and extreme fatigue are early signs of deficiency.

Food sources of Potassium

If you eat a lot of processed foods, the important balance between sodium and potassium is not achieved, since most processed foods contain large amounts of sodium. This is one more reason why it is very important to avoid processed foods in general. Potassium is found in potatoes, spinach, mushrooms, broccoli, dates, bananas, avocado, lucuma and nuts.

Sodium

The Details

-Sodium works with potassium to help muscle contraction and expansion. It also works with potassium for stimulating nerves (20).

-Sodium is involved in oxygen transport.

-It is necessary for making hydrochloric acid in the digestive track, so it helps to break down food and keep digestion smooth.

-Too much sodium can cause you to lose a lot of potassium in the urine, potentially leading to potassium deficiency.

-The quality of sodium that is in processed foods is very bad. Use sea salt whenever possible.

-Fluids need to be replaced before sodium, because sodium can't be absorbed without liquids (20).

Signs of Sodium Deficiency

Deficiency is very unusual in the United States. It is more likely you would have too much than too little. However, if you sweat a lot and eat almost no processed foods whatsoever you may need to add more salt to you diet. Also, if you never take in any electrolytes but drink a ton of water, you run the risk of water intoxication. Water intoxication occurs when the balance of electrolytes in the body is outside of a safe range, and can be very dangerous. See the chapter on hydration to make sure you are hydrated and keeping your electrolytes in check. Not having enough sodium can also lead to heart palpitations, muscle weakness and shrinking of the muscles (20).

Food sources of Sodium

Sea salt, kelp

Sulfur

The Details

-Sulfur is a part of protein molecules (20).

-It is necessary for synthesis of collagen (20).

-It helps keep skin, nails and hair in good shape.

-It is found in insulin.

-Sulfur plays a part in the process where oxygen and other substances are used to build cells and release energy (20).

-Sulfur can be helpful in treating arthritis.

-MSM contains sulfur.

-It can help skin issues when used topically.

Signs of Sulfur Deficiency

Though there are no clear signs of sulfur deficiency, I would speculate that constant muscle soreness and joint discomfort are probably your body's way of telling you that you need some more sulfur.

Food sources

Beans

Trace minerals

Chromium

The Details

-Chromium is needed for metabolizing carbohydrates and fats.

-Chromium stimulates fatty acid and cholesterol synthesis, which are important for brain function and other body processes.[28]

-Chromium is important in the breakdown of insulin.

Signs of Chromium Deficiency

-A chromium deficiency typically shows up in the form of the body being unable to process glucose well.[29] Deficiency is more common in people who engage in regular strenuous exercise (20).

Food sources of Chromium

Wheat germ, green peppers, apples, banana, spinach, black pepper, and molasses

Copper

The Details

-Copper plays a role in respiration.

-Copper is involved in the production of collagen and the neurotransmitter noradrenalin (20). Noradrenalin is a "fight or flight" chemical.

-Copper helps cell membranes remain healthy.

-Copper helps the body form red blood cells.

---

[28] http://www.nlm.nih.gov/medlineplus/ency/article/002418.htm

[29] http://www.nlm.nih.gov/medlineplus/ency/article/002418.htm

[30] http://www.nlm.nih.gov/medlineplus/ency/article/002419.htm

-Copper keeps the blood vessels, immune system, nerves, and bones healthy.[30]

-It aids healing processes (20).

-It is needed to synthesize substances that are used to form the myelin sheaths surrounding nerve fibers (20). Remember how important myelin is in perfecting athletic movements!

-It works with vitamin C to form Elastin, which is a big part of the elastic connective tissue found all over the body (20).

-An imbalance of copper and zinc can cause issues with the thyroid (20).

Signs of Copper Deficiency

Anemia, osteoporosis, impaired respiration, easily damaged connective tissue, bone and joint issues (20)

Food sources of Copper:

Whole grains, beans, nuts, potatoes, dark leafy greens, dried fruits, cacao, black pepper, thyme, paprika, bay leaves (20)

Fluoride

The Details

-Fluoride stimulates formation of bone and helps prevent tooth decay. Bones and teeth have a crystalline structure that is strengthened by fluoride (20).

Signs of Fluoride Deficiency

Deficiency is very rare in the US, but excessive amounts are very harmful, since they can destroy enzymes.

Food sources of Fluoride

Sea vegetables are the best source, but fluoride is also found in kidney beans, lettuce, and spinach (20).

Iodine

The Details

-Iodine is needed for normal thyroid function and metabolism of cells.

-It is needed for the production of thyroid hormones.[31]

-It can be lost through perspiration (20)

Signs of Iodine Deficiency

Without enough iodine, thyroid cells and the thyroid gland get enlarged (31). Other signs of deficiency include fatigue, cold intolerance, rapid pulse, heart palpitations, dry hair and skin, nervousness, and irritability (20).

Food sources of Iodine

Kelp and other sea vegetables, foods grown in iodine rich soil (31)

---

[31] http://www.nlm.nih.gov/medlineplus/ency/article/002421.htm

Iron

The Details

-Iron is needed to make the oxygen-carrying proteins hemoglobin and myoglobin.

-It makes up part of many proteins in the body.[32]

-It plays a role in transportation of oxygen from lungs to body tissue (20).

-It returns carbon dioxide from tissues to lungs.

-Too much iron can be toxic if you don't need it, and the body can only get rid of iron through blood loss. It is therefore not advisable to take an iron supplement unless there are circumstances that cause you to have low iron levels: for example if you have a very heavy menstrual flow or if you have tested for low iron levels. Children have different iron needs than adults, so it is best to check with your health care provider about whether or not they should be supplementing with iron and, if so, how much (24).

-As Dr. Weil cautions, "Iron is an oxidizing agent-the sort of thing antioxidants protect us from-and too much in the body can promote unhealthy changes in cells, increasing risks of cardiovascular disease and cancer." (24)

-Vitamin C helps you to absorb Iron better (24).

Signs of Iron Deficiency

Lack of energy, shortness of breath, headaches, irritability, and anemia.

Food sources

Dried beans, dried fruits, whole grains, almonds, broccoli, spinach, kale,

[32] http://www.nlm.nih.gov/medlineplus/ency/article/002422.htm

collards, asparagus, dandelion greens, millet, oats, brown rice, and cacao.

Manganese

The Details

-It helps metabolize protein, carbohydrate, and fat.

-It helps regulate blood sugar (20).

-It helps bones develop.

-It helps form blood and collagen.

-It helps digest protein.

-It contributes to proper functioning of the immune system.

-It helps activate enzymes involved in energy production.

-It helps protect cells from damage and inflammation.

- Since Manganese can stimulate the transmission of impulses between the nerves and muscles, it has been used in combination with B vitamins to help people who suffer from terrible muscle weakness (20).

Signs of Manganese Deficiency

Glucose intolerance can be a sign that there is a manganese deficiency. There has also been a connection between diets deficient in manganese and incidence of loss of muscle control. Sometimes dizziness, ear noises, and loss of hearing can be traced back to a manganese deficiency (20).

Dietary sources of Manganese

Nuts, whole grains, dried fruits, green leafy veggies, brown rice, lentils, pineapple, blackberries, sweet potato and persimmons are all good sources of manganese. It is important to know that the amounts of manganese found in these foods can vary due to soil being stripped of this mineral by ammonia fertilizers.

Molybdenum

The Details

-It is required for three important enzyme systems (20).

-It helps detoxify sulfites.

Signs of Molybdenum Deficiency

Excessive amounts of sulfites in the body, headaches, rapid breathing or asthma, visual problems (20)

Food sources of Molybdenum

Legumes, dark leafy green vegetables, soybeans, oatmeal, and cauliflower

Selenium

The Details

-Selenium behaves primarily as an antioxidant.

-It helps keep skin elasticity.

-It prevents hardening of the arteries.

-It deals with changes in hormone production and hormone receptors.

-It helps repair DNA.

-It boosts immune function.

-It can decrease inflammation and improve strength and vigor (20).

-In the blood, it has anti-clotting affects.

-It can improve energy and mood (20).

Signs of Selenium Deficiency:

Premature aging, heart disease, skin problems/irritations, inflammation, fertility issues

Food sources of Selenium

Brazil nuts, mushrooms

Zinc

The Details

-It is a part of more than 200 enzymes and therefore helps with digestion of protein, production of energy, and absorption of vitamins, among other things (20).

-It fights disease.

-It protects the immune system.

-It helps the activities of many hormones (20).

-It helps heal wounds and shorten colds (20).

-It is good for Rheumatoid Arthritis symptoms and diseases where inflammation is a factor (20).

Signs of Zinc Deficiency

Athletes who don't eat a lot of zinc or eat too many processed foods are at risk of being deficient since sweating carries zinc away from the body. People who don't have enough zinc tend to get chronic infections and kidney disease. It is really important to get zinc while you are growing since a lack of zinc can cause slow growth (20). Other signs of deficiency include skin problems, decreased taste and smell, fatigue, unusual menstrual periods, poor circulation, and the tendency to faint (20).

Food sources of Zinc

Pumpkin seeds, legumes, wheat germ, and whole grains are all good sources of Zinc. Once again, however, you won't get a lot of Zinc in your diet if these foods were grown in nutrient-poor soil.

So hopefully, now you are acquainted with the different micronutrients, what they do, and how you can eat them. You are probably noticing that leafy green vegetables come up quite frequently when I list "Food sources of . . ." This is not a coincidence as these are the foods that you should be eating the most. The take-home message from this chapter is that taking a few nutrients in pill form can make you worse in the long run instead of better. On the other hand, if you are always eating nutrient-dense unrefined foods, you don't really have to worry much about whether or not you have enough micronutrients on board to both protect your health and support your athletic endeavors. Dr. Fuhrman definitely summarized it best:

> It may never be possible to extract the precise symphony of nutrients found in vegetation and place it in a pill. Isolated nutrients extracted from food may never offer the same level of disease-protective effects of whole natural foods, as nature 'designed them.' Fruits and vegetables contain a variety of nutrients, which work in subtle synergies, and many of these nutrients cannot be isolated or extracted. Phytochemicals from a variety of plant foods work together to become much more potent at detoxifying carcinogens and protecting against cancer than when

taken individually as isolated compounds. [33]

---

[33] Fuhrman, Joel. (2011). Eat to Live: The Amazing Nutrient-Rich Program for Fast and Sustained Weight Loss (revised edition). New York. Little, Brown and Company.

CHAPTER FOUR:
BUSTING MACRONUTRIENT MYTHS

Every few years, a newly packaged version of a high-protein diet comes out. Carbohydrates are depicted as some sort of nefarious villain that has been sabotaging weight loss efforts for your entire life! High protein diets are always touted as an easy way to lose weight and get into shape. Lots of people buy into them, lose weight temporarily, and then inevitability put the weight back on.

First and foremost, you should be wary of any diet that demonizes one particular group of macronutrients (macronutrients are protein, carbohydrates and fats). The truth is, that your body needs protein, carbohydrates and fats to function optimally. Athletes, in particular, need fats and carbohydrates because fats and carbohydrates are optimal sources of fuel for activity. Of course, the types of fats and carbohydrates you choose are extremely important, but more on that later.

I think that high protein diets tend to always gain popularity because most people think: "surely, you can't possibly get too much protein, right?"

Not quite.

Nutritionist and RD Elizabeth Somer stated that most Americans get two to three times more protein than they need. Too much of this nutrient leads your body to turn the excess into acids that stress your kidneys and liver.[34]

If you eat more protein than you need, the body burns it for fuel. Protein molecules are extremely complex, and your body therefore uses a lot of energy to take them apart and metabolize them. Eating a lot of protein is therefore a pretty inefficient fuel source when compared to fat and carbohydrates if you are prepping for competition. Basically, if you eat a huge meatball sandwich before you compete, your body can either break down that protein or expend energy trying to achieve optimum athletic success, but it certainly cannot do both.

The other problem with protein as a fuel source is that it doesn't burn very cleanly. Fats and carbohydrates release only carbon dioxide and water as they are burned (24). Protein on the other hand, leaves a nitrogen-containing residue in the form of ammonia when it is burned. Ammonia, as you might already be aware, is toxic, and the body needs to eliminate it. Eating too much protein can therefore actually place a lot of added stress on the liver and kidneys and is also a lot more work for the digestive system (24). The body has to convert ammonia into urea, which is eliminated by the kidneys. Increased production of urea stresses the kidneys, but also creates a need for water loss in the urine to remove ammonia from the body. This diuretic effect as a result of eating too much protein has the consequence of removing minerals from the body, especially calcium: "It is well known that high-protein diets promote calcium loss and so increase the risk of osteoporosis, the common condition of weakened bones . . . " (Dr.

---

[34] Fontoura, Maria. (2014, April 20). Diet Like a Man. *Health*. 39-45.

Weil, 24)

Dr. Weil has also hypothesized that high-protein diets can aggravate the immune system, leaving it more likely to react to harmless substances in the environment (allergies) or go after the body's own tissues (autoimmune conditions). This is definitely a very strong theory since casein, the protein in milk, is known to set off allergies. In fact, he advises anyone with autoimmune issues to limit the amount of protein consumed (24).

You might think that, based on the information above, I have some gripe with protein.

This could not be further from the truth. Protein is very important, particularly as a part of the recovery process for an athlete. The body uses it to repair damaged tissues, build muscle, and maintain optimal functioning. I just want to make you aware of the dangers of eating *too much* of it. So what is too much protein? Most people can't digest more than 26 grams in a sitting. For vegans and vegetarians, we really don't have to worry much about going over that number. If you are an omnivore, however, it can be very easy to go over that number, so be mindful.

So is it possible to get *too little* protein? It's really only possible if your diet is high in processed and refined foods and low in green vegetables. In that case, you are also in danger of not getting many vital nutrients and fiber. Unprocessed plant foods contain carbohydrates, proteins, and fats. Approximately 25 percent of the calories in vegetables come from protein (33). Additionally, 100 calories of broccoli actually has MORE protein than 100 calories of sirloin steak (33). You will not be protein-deficient if you eat a lot of green vegetables and have variety in your diet. Beans, nuts, seeds and quinoa are also great sources of protein. Athletes, of course, need more protein than the average person, but they also need to consume more calories in general. As you consume more calories from green vegetables, fruits, seeds, nuts and a few other superfoods, you will automatically get enough of what you need (33). No more counting grams of protein, fat, or calories. Ahhh, freedom.

Even if you are an omnivore and plan on staying that way (I still love you, don't worry), you would do well to get more of your protein from plant sources. Dr. Fuhrman recommends that 90 percent of calories should come from unrefined plant foods (33), even if you do eat meat. Vegetarians and vegans who primarily consume processed and industrialized foods are really no better off than their omnivorous counterparts. Plant protein from whole, unrefined, plant foods is for everyone. It has enormous implications for health and performance in the addition to the following advantages:

-Plant protein is less perishable than meat.

-Plant protein is less likely to have high concentrations of environmental toxins because plants are lower on the food chain.

-The fat that generally accompanies plant protein is better for you than animal fat.

-Plant protein contains fiber and micronutrients that animal foods lack. Fiber slows down the absorption of glucose and helps to control the speed of digestion. If you think that you can just get more fiber from the fiber that is added to industrialized "foods," then you are mistaken. That fiber is often sourced from bamboo or similar fibers that are not really good for you. You need to eat high-fiber foods instead of adding fiber supplements in order to get its anti-carcinogenic benefits and the benefits of all the other nutrients in the plant (33).

-The protein in vegetables is less concentrated, so you can eat more without overloading system with protein (24).

-Nutritional energy starts out as solar energy that green plants gather and store by using photosynthesis. This process generates one of the most basic foods for cells of plants and animals. It is the "fuel that many cells prefer to use in order to obtain energy" (24). If you are eating the animal, you are basically getting the nutrition of the plants through a filtration device.

-The idea that plant foods don't contain all of the proteins we need is a myth.[35]

-Research is beginning to show that many degenerative diseases have their origin in an animal-focused dietary approach (35).

-Almost all plant foods (including berries) have at least some protein.

-Plant foods are alkaline forming, while animal foods are acid forming. Too much acid in the body can inhibit recovery and promote growth of bad things (like cancer).

So does this mean that you should go dive head first into a bowl full of oatmeal? Well, no, not really. Most of your diet should really be composed of organic green vegetables. But know that carbohydrates are not the enemy, it is the quality and quantity of carbohydrates that are consumed that pack on extra pounds and make us sluggish.

The fact is, we are far too reliant on processed and industrialized carbohydrates. We eat a lot of wheat, which has been so crossbred throughout the history of farming that it doesn't even resemble the wheat that our ancestors ate. Corn, technically a grain, has also been crossbreed to a point where it is nearly unrecognizable from its original form. We have made it so that it is sweeter and much less nutritionally dense.[36] So what's an athlete to do for good sources of carbohydrates?

---

[35] (2014 March). Nutrition Matters: Separating Trends from Fads. *IDEA Fitness Journal, 11(3)*, 36-43.

[36] Robinson, Jo. (2013). *Eating on the Wild Side.* New York: Little Brown, and Co.

Let's keep it simple: the best sources of carbohydrates will be fruits and vegetables. Period. Pseudograins are another good source of carbohydrates, but should not be used as frequently as fruits and vegetables. Pseudograins are technically seeds that are used like grains. They are also typically a pretty good source of protein. Amaranth, buckwheat and quinoa are all pseudograins and all excellent sources of phytonutrients, vitamins, and minerals. Finally, grains should only be a very small part of your carbohydrate intake. Brown rice, black rice, red rice, teff, steel-cut oats, kamut, millet, sorghum, barley, and corn are all grains and should be used sparingly and only in their whole-foods state (never processed). For example, if you do eat wheat, it should only ever be sprouted wheat with pretty much no preservatives. So your daily carbohydrate consumption should look something like this:

Grains

Pseudograins

Fresh, whole fruits

Starchy Vegetables: tubers, carrots, sweet potatoes

Green vegetables such as kale, chard, spinach, broccoli, arugula, etc.

Notice in the pyramid, that most of your carbohydrates should come from green vegetables (peas do not count as they are technically a legume) and the least amount of carbohydrates should come from grains of any sort. Notice that "sugar" is not in the pyramid. Added sugars can be very inflammatory and also addicting. I therefore think that all individuals, but especially athletes who should be very concerned about how much inflammation is occurring in their bodies, should really not put any added sugar in their diets. Fruit is plenty sweet when it is organic and in-season.

For those of you wondering where mushrooms fall on this pyramid, mushrooms are actually neither vegetables nor plants. We have more DNA sequences in common with mushrooms than we do with plants. They contain some protein along with trace minerals and vitamins. They are also immunity enhancers (24). I personally eat as many mushrooms as I want, particularly Shitake and Portobello. My new favorite is actually Trumpet mushrooms. Mushrooms should always be cooked prior to eating.

So why do carbohydrates get such a bad rap? Well, once we process them, we take out all of the micronutrients and fiber and fill it with chemicals. Just as a quick example of something that has been approved by the FDA to go into food and cosmetics (this is directly from Dr. Weil's book):

FD7C(food, drug and cosmetic) Yellow No.6 (sunset yellow)- This has been shown to cause allergic reactions like hives, rhinitis (runny nose) and nasal congestion. It appeared to cause tumors of the kidney and adrenal glands in rats, and it may be carcinogenic. The FDA reviewed studies on rats and believes that this color is safe to use. This color is banned in Norway and Sweden. It has been found used in sausages, candy gelatin, and baked goods.

(24)

That is just the tip of the iceberg. There is some pretty scary stuff in processed food (and I do count "whole wheat" bread as a processed food). In fact, introducing processed and western foods to cultures with traditional diets has increased their rates of obesity and disease. Not surprisingly, studies done with Hawaiians and O'odham who were having health issues showed that, when they began eating their traditional carbohydrate staples, their health problems improved. A traditional Hawaiian diet incorporates poi, breadfruit, and sweet potatoes. A traditional O'odham diet incorporates beans, squash, and corn. None of the foods mentioned are low in carbohydrates, but they do have a low glycemic index and can be eaten in a whole foods state (unprocessed, unrefined). This is an important study, because it reinforces the idea that it is the *kind* of carbohydrate you eat (read: unprocessed) that is critical (24). Just like protein, however, the *amount* of carbohydrate you eat is also important. You should not have much more than 60 grams in a sitting, because it is difficult for your body to use more than that. This number can be very easy to surpass if you eat a lot of fruits and/or grains in one sitting, but it is very difficult to surpass if you eat a lot of leafy green vegetables.

Another myth to tackle is the idea that you cannot eat fat with carbohydrate. Again, it has to do with the quality of carbohydrate and fat. Fat in a food actually brings down glycemic index by slowing down how fast the stomach empties. It therefore also slows down the digestion of the starch (24).

Speaking of fats . . . . .

Fats are so complicated. There is so much drama around these macronutrient divas. Probably no other macronutrient is as highly debated as fats. If you feel like you want to run screaming from the room every time someone brings up "healthy fats," you are not alone. There are trans fats, saturated fats, Omega 3s, Omega 6s, EFAs, oh my!

It is almost like fats are being deliberately confusing.

The truth is, we really NEED fats. Proponents of low-fat and no fat diets must have missed the memo about something called EFAs: that stands for Essential Fatty Acids, and your body can't produce them on its own, so you absolutely have to consume them in food. Linolenic and linoleic acid are essential fatty acids. If your body doesn't get enough of these, you can have depression, dry skin, sub-optimal functioning of the immune system, and problems with the liver and kidneys. Linolenic and linoleic acid are used to build Omega 3s and Omega 6s. The problem is Omega-6s and Omega-3s compete with each other to get used in the body. So your ratio for consuming them should be 1:1. However, most Americans eat more like 10:1 Omega 6 to Omega 3 or even 25:1. Yikes! This can be bad for inflammation and other important functions in the body, particularly since Omega-3s play a huge role in forming cell walls throughout the body. They also help circulation and oxygen uptake. So why are our ratios of Omega-3s to Omega-6s so skewed? This is, once again, a result of a diet very high in processed foods.[37]

So now, everyone wants to get those Omega-3s. This explains everyone's obsession with fish oil. There are Omega-3s in fish oil, but only because fish eat lots of sea vegetables. Soooo, if *you* eat lots of sea vegetables you are basically cutting out the middleman (or middlefish, as the case may be). On the plant side of things, flaxseeds, walnuts, chia seeds, hemp seeds, and certain leafy greens are all good sources of Omega-3s.

So how do we simplify these complicated fats?

All the fats that come from plants are extremely good for you until they are heated or processed. Many oils become unstable at high temperatures and are therefore not healthy to consume. Vegetable oils are often extracted with heat, chemical solvents, and pressure. This can create trans-fatty acids. These are very bad. Also, don't ever eat anything with hydrogenated fats in it (24). This leads us to the point that you should basically never eat anything deep-fried. Ever. That oil is unstable after heating it just once, but, having worked at a concession stand, I know that they only change that oil about once a week. If that isn't gross enough to make you swear off the sauce, just think about all of the free radicals that those bad fats are creating in your body. Stay away!

---

[37] http://www.pcrm.org/health/health-topics/essential-fatty-acids

Here are some great sources of fats:

-avocados

-flax seeds

-chia seeds

-hemp seeds

-pumpkin seeds

-sesame seeds

-coconuts

-nuts

Just as one more incentive to make your diet more heavily plant-based, vegetarians have much higher levels of stored EFAs than omnivores (24).

So I know you are probably thinking, "well what do I cook with then?" I would suggest using mostly coconut oil and olive oil, but again, try not to make the temperatures super high or use too much oil. Oil, even coconut and olive oil, doesn't have all the nutrients and phytonutrients of the whole food (i.e. the whole olive or coconut). Oil has very few nutrients other than some vitamin E, so you are always better off consuming food in its whole form (33).

Even though you should currently have a pretty good idea about some great sources for micronutrients and macronutrients, you still might not have the perfect diet for you. Why? Food sensitivities are very common and can cause you to feel run down, lethargic, congested, and moody. They can also cause stomach pain, migraines, and a lot of other symptoms that can hinder your performance. Many people with food sensitivities have difficulty losing weight even after making appropriate changes to their diets. Food sensitivities are different from allergies. Allergies generally show up in testing and if you have a severe allergy, exposure can sometimes be life-threatening. Sensitivities are often more subtle in terms of how they manifest, but can really make you feel miserable. So here are some common troublemakers:

Soy

Wheat

Dairy

Corn

Preservatives/chemicals/dyes in processed foods

Artificial sweeteners

Yeast

Caffeine

Peanuts

If you just looked at "caffeine" and then wanted to choke me for putting it on the list: a) you probably drink too much caffeine and b) we will discuss caffeine more in the chapter on hydration. There is a lot of conflicting information out there about it, particularly for athletes. Your consumption of caffeine really affects your hydration, so we will discuss it more thoroughly later. If you need your caffeine fix now, skip ahead.

As far as the other items on the above list are concerned, the best way to determine whether or not you actually do have food sensitivities is to do an elimination diet. There are a few different ways to accomplish this, so do your homework and find out what is best for you. Typically, you would eliminate one potential offender for two weeks or more and see how you feel. If you suddenly feel great, don't chalk it up to coincidence. Alternatively, some people like to eliminate all of items mentioned above for at least two weeks and then introduce the items back into the diet one at a time over a series of several weeks. Try what feels right for you and works with your schedule. At this point, you shouldn't be eating any processed foods or artificial sweeteners anyway, since you would probably get about the same nutrition from noshing on a piece of cardboard (with less risk of cancer). That should make eliminating food dyes and chemicals a bit easier. When you do your elimination diet, just be aware that soy, wheat, corn, and dairy are in almost everything, so you have to read labels. If you are food sensitive, sometimes even small amounts of the offending substance can make you feel subpar, so be thorough if you are going to try an elimination diet.

I used to get terrible heartburn and migranes, but when I cut out dairy and wheat completely, I couldn't believe how great I felt. People are often surprised to find that dairy is typically very bad for health, since we associate it with getting calcium. The calcium in dairy, however, is really not utilized as effectively as the calcium in plants because dairy makes the body very acidic. Additionally, we lose the enzymes to break dairy down as we age and casein is known to set off allergies and immune responses. For those of you who are scratching your head and wondering how to milk a broccoli floret, you can put your mind at ease. Just by eating lots of broccoli and other whole plant foods, you will be getting calcium that is very easy to digest and won't make your body acidic.

What?

Yes, another great upside to having a diet that is primarily plant-based is that pretty much everything you eat will be alkaline-forming. Eating alkaline-forming foods helps your body to recover faster and get sick less frequently. Examples of alkaline foods would be mustard greens, apples, spinach, and almost all fruits and vegetables. On the other hand, processed foods such as soda, meats, and dairy are examples of foods that make your body very acidic. Eating acid-forming foods on a regular basis causes your body to attempt to maintain a reasonable PH by leaching calcium from your bones to return to an alkaline state. Over time, this contributes to fatigue, sub-par performance, and chronic inflammation. Watch your recovery time improve as you start adding more alkaline foods to your diet.

So for those of you who are still thinking that a whole-foods, primarily plant-based diet is not the way to go, here are some other things you will only find in plants:

Antioxidants

Here's something you'll never hear: "Berries? No thank you, I just got all of the antioxidants I'll need out of that steak." Antioxidants can stop or slow down damage that is a result of oxygen. The term "antioxidant" therefore reflects a chemical property and includes certain vitamins, minerals, and phytochemicals. Antioxidants are found mostly in fruits and veggies.[38]

Phytonutrients

Even if you have never heard the term "phytonutrients," I am sure that you are familiar with some of the "A-listers" from this group that hog all the attention. Some very popular phytonutrients are lycopene, beta-carotene, resveratrol, quercetin, allicin, and capsaicin, but there are literally

---

[38] http://www.medterms.com/script/main/art.asp?articlekey=11291

1000s of phytonutrients. So what are these wonderful little gems? Phytonutrients are the naturally occurring chemicals in plants that help protect the plants from germs, fungus, and other potential threats at survival. When we consume them, they help us to prevent disease and keep the body functioning optimally. So as you begin incorporating more plant foods, don't be fooled by clever advertising. Some supplement companies are isolating phytonutrients and then marketing them as a way to solve all of your problems. Remember from the previous chapter, however, that taking resveratrol in a capsule is not the same as getting it in a food.[39]

Polysaccharides

The type of polysaccharides specifically found in mushrooms (not button mushrooms, but shiitake and oyster) (24) appear to be the component of certain medicinal plants that can boost immunity and help destroy malignant cells.

Nitrates

For those of you who recognize this as something that is in hotdogs and are currently thinking: "ah-ha, finally! A reason to eat hot dogs!" I am so sorry to disappoint (not really). The nitrates I am referring to are in beets and beet juice, and they help the muscles use oxygen more efficiently. They can also help to improve circulation. Getting back to hotdogs, nitrate and nitrite are added to cured meats as a preservative. There has been some speculation that when they are heated they come together with another

---

[39] http://www.webmd.com/diet/phytonutrients-faq

[40] http://www.theglobeandmail.com/life/health-and-fitness/fitness/why-elite-athletes-guzzle-beet-juice-before-a-race/article12747831/

group of chemicals found in cured meats that could produce carcinogens. The nitrates found naturally occurring in vegetables, however, are very safe as long as they are not taken in supplement form (eat, instead of taking a pill, for goodness sake!). Some other plant sources of nitrate are arugula, rhubarb, celery, and swiss chard. For those of you thinking that this has no relevance to athletic performance, there was a study that went so far as to prove that people who ate beets prior to a run we able to run faster than those in the control group.[40]

Finally, a lot of substances that occur naturally in plant foods have been shown to be anti-carcinogenic. Again, these substances do not work well as isolated compounds, but rather, work holistically when you eat the plant. Allium compounds, catechins, ellagic acid, flavonoids, isoflavones, phenolic acids, protease inhibitors, and sterols are literally just a few examples. This list can go on and on (33).

So take that, naysayers!

Keep in mind, if this is all new information to you, don't feel compelled to make a million changes at once. In fact, if all you have ever eaten is meat and you try to go plant-based overnight, all of the extra fiber might make your roommates hate you. Do only as much as you can handle, and as you start to feel better, make your diet cleaner and cleaner. There are going to be setbacks with any nutrition plan, but do the best you can within your means. It's not easy at first, but eventually you won't crave any of the garbage anymore.

Here are some things to keep in mind:

-Processed foods and caffeine are designed to be addicting. As you wean yourself off of them, don't be surprised if you experience some withdrawal symptoms. This may include some headaches, fatigue and hunger at first.

Go at your own pace. Gradually you will feel better and better.

-You are currently accustomed to eating large quantities of meat and bread, so it will take you some time to get used to eating HUGE portions of leafy green vegetables. You have to do a lot of chewing and have to actually plan to sit down and eat! Pick an organic dressing that you really enjoy and use it to enhance the flavors of your veggies. I have a serious hummus addiction and I will pretty much use any vegetable imaginable to spoon it in my mouth.

-Things that excite your taste buds now will be disgusting to you a year from now. If your favorite restaurant is currently McDonald's (aka Satan), or you can't imagine ever not liking Dunkin' Donuts (a minion), you will be surprised how that food tastes like chemicals and crap (which is basically what it is) once you start eating real food. Don't expect it to happen overnight. I used to be really addicted to sweet things and now I find that I really can't eat more than a bite of anything that is sweeter than fruit. Dark chocolate: that's a different story.

-You are probably about to lose some weight. Don't get concerned! Your body will naturally regulate after a while. When I first became vegan, I lost so much weight that my mom was concerned, but over time, I started to gain it back and got more energy, strength and endurance.

Okay, so now you know what to eat, and what not to eat, so the next important question becomes: when?

CHAPTER FIVE:
(NUTRIENT) TIMING IS EVERYTHING

In case you haven't figured this out already, I am a bit of a bookworm. I read EVERYTHING, and have therefore read an insane amount of material on nutrient timing. Plus, I have taken courses, been to lectures, and generally soaked up every piece of information I could.

After dissecting all of this information, I definitely think that optimal nutrient timing requires some planning and can vary somewhat depending on what time of day your training is. If you train twice a day, that might complicate things further. For example, working out first thing in the morning creates an entirely different set of circumstances then if you work out after dinner (which is not preferable, if you can help it). Additionally, I do think there is *some* need for individual tailoring (though the basic concepts apply to all athletes). I believe that taking the best that research has to offer and then customizing it to suit your own individual body and preferences is pretty much the way to go for in all things in life. So keep that in mind as you are reading this chapter. Yes, I am a bit of a tree-hugging hippy, but this isn't about "we are all beautiful snowflakes." It is simply anatomy and microbiology. If I weigh 100 pounds and am competing as a top gymnast, I am not going to have the same nutrient needs as a marathoner or an Olympic weight lifter.

The food you put into your body prior to competition should not be the same as what you put in during, which is also different from what you should be eating after your workout. This is something that most athletes don't know, but it can make a huge difference in performance. Here are the things that will best improve your performance and recovery in all the stages of competition:

Prior to your workout/game: In general, your body will need high quality carbohydrates and fats to burn during competition. I stress the phase "high quality" here. If you are thinking that a whole-wheat bagel with cream cheese is okay before competition, then you need to go back and re-read the first few chapters. Instead of going for processed garbage, try to use carbohydrates and fats that are super-foods or at least as nutrient-dense as possible.

It is also really important to plan for how much time you have before the game or workout. If you have two hours or more before your competition, you can eat a high quality "mixed meal." A mixed meal would consist of all of the macronutrients (protein, carbohydrates, and fats). You just have to be careful to avoid overloading your system with vegetables here, since you don't want to get gassy on the court, field, etc. Know how much you are capable of eating without discomfort and plan from there. I wouldn't really plan on a rice and beans dish with onions and broccoli if I were you. Nope, save that for a first date that you hope will not become a second.

If your competition is in the morning and you like to sleep until the last possible second, then you should be eating something really simple like a banana with almond butter. For goodness sake, no bacon, egg and cheese! For those of you who get some butterflies before an athletic performance, then you want to eat a small, easily digestible snack. The same rules apply if you are trying to fuel while you have a short break in between games. A huge mistake that I have seen numerous athletes make is consuming an entire sandwich and a bag of chips seconds before going out to play a game. Your body can either digest that sandwich or perform, but it cannot do both. This leaves many athletes in a difficult situation, since sometimes you can be at the field or on the court all day and you are definitely going to need sustenance during that time. This is where planning and packing a few things makes all the difference.

Digestibility is always a very important characteristic of the food you consume on game day, but even more so if you are eating quickly in between games. If you just finished a game and have to perform in another one immediately after, don't stop and get a turkey sandwich. Your body is going to have to work so hard to digest that protein that you will be detracting from your performance. Instead, stick with something like a high-quality energy bar (different from a protein bar, make sure you read the labels!), fruit, nuts, seeds, or maybe some (barely processed or raw) organic granola.

If you have a game early on in the day and you are sleeping at home (as opposed to traveling), a terrific breakfast would be fermented steel cut oats with berries and almond butter. The fermentation increases digestibility of the oats and cuts way down on cooking time. Fermenting also allows some healthy bacteria to grow. The oats are a great source of complex carbohydrates and the almond butter is a terrific source of fat. You can also add a little coconut oil for some additional energy (as fat). The berries are filled with antioxidants, micronutrients and great flavor. If this combination is not sweet enough, you can add a little maple syrup. This is an ideal breakfast, but unrealistic if you are traveling or if you have to be at the field at 6AM. In these instances, you need something that is easy to carry and provides maximum nutrition while your body expends minimal energy on digestion. A good example is a piece of fruit and a handful of nuts. If you do a little planning, you can soak two tablespoons of chia seeds and three tablespoons of hemp seed in almond or coconut milk the night before your game. Leave it in the refrigerator overnight, and then breakfast is ready for you when you wake up. Some people refer to this as "chia pudding." Soaking the seeds makes them easier to digest and they are a great source of fat. Add a banana, apple, some berries, or melon to the mix and you have a pre-game super-food snack! This mix travels very well in a Pyrex container with an ice pack. You can eat it in the car on the way to the field or court.

This is that part during my seminars (for more on my seminars and workshops, flip to the back of the book) in which someone invariably stops me, incredulous, and asks "what about protein?" Many people are not aware of the fact that most fruits, vegetables, grains, and pseudo-grains do contain at least some protein, and you will definitely not become deficient in a matter of hours. Remember, as a rule, we all actually tend to over-consume protein. Additionally, when you are out there in competition, your body is not burning protein (we hope!), and, unless you have a history of disordered eating, you are not going to run out of protein in a day's worth of games. Protein intake is really essential in the recovery phase, but not during the game. As someone who has been a personal trainer for over 10 years now, this information came as a shock at first. Personal trainers as a population tend to consume ridiculous amounts of protein. It is actually a bit outlandish. When I first became certified, I always used to load up on protein before games, while staying around 20 grams of carbohydrates. I would then wonder why I was feeling sluggish and hungry by the fifth inning. The reason is simple: your body needs to burn fat and carbohydrates while it is working out, so those are the best things to consume prior to competition. Plus, if you remember from the earlier chapters, fat helps the carbohydrates to burn more slowly, so you won't be starving when it counts. That having been addressed, there are times when I do go for a little extra protein before workouts, just based on what I am craving and how I am feeling. As long as there is not an absurd amount of protein, and the emphasis is still on high quality fats and carbohydrates, I don't think your performance will suffer much.

Immediately following your workout/game: It is very important that you replenish depleted glycogen stores within thirty minutes of finishing competition. This is an important piece of optimal recovery. Most athletes think that protein is really important here, but you really only want a small amount. You actually want a 4:1 carbohydrate to protein ratio (four grams of carbohydrate for every one gram of protein). Eating more protein than that can actually have a negative effect. It slows rehydration and glycogen replenishment. If you are currently thinking "there is no way I am doing this kind of math after competition," you are not alone! I always like to keep my post-workout simple and just have some Vega Recovery Accelerator after an extremely strenuous workout. I am not sponsored or in any way endorsed by Vega (though I would love to be: take the hint, Vega!), but I do find their products absolutely superior to anything on the market. They also have a very important feature for us as athletes. They carry the "Informed Choice" Certification. What does this mean? Since supplements are not FDA regulated and can carry all sorts of nasty things that can test you positive for drugs (that's right: scary stuff). An "Informed Choice" Certification, "assures athletes that products carrying the INFORMED-CHOICE mark have been regularly tested for substances considered prohibited in sport. In addition, INFORMED-CHOICE also ensures that products have been manufactured to high quality standards."[41] You should be seeing this label on ALL the supplements you are using: otherwise you might be unwittingly putting your eligibility at risk.

But what if you don't want to purchase Vega or if you want to chew your calories? Some cacao nibs and a handful of goji berries put you in about the right ratio. I am also a huge fan of seaweed chips after workouts, but I am realistic and understand that most people think this is pretty gross. On practice days and hard training days, you can experiment with different types of portable snacks, so you know exactly what works best for you on game day. I personally really like salty stuff after working out (or things that contain salt naturally, like celery with some kind of great dip), but there are times when I work out so hard I can't even think about putting something in my mouth afterwards. I just listen to my body and respect it when that happens. I will wait until I feel ready to eat, regardless of the time frame. I am very rarely sore, so I don't think this impedes my progress very much.

Most of the time you will just be having a snack within 30 minutes of

---

[41] www.informed-choice.org

finishing your workouts/competitions, but if you finish late at night and you won't be awake for very long after competition, you will probably want to have a mixed meal instead of just a snack. I also think it is a good idea to eat a mixed meal right after competition if you are starving. It makes no sense to have just a snack and wait a full two hours for a meal if you are really hungry. Plus, if you are finishing late at night, you don't really want to stay awake any longer than you have to. I pitched a game at a tournament once where we finished well after midnight and had an early game the next morning. I didn't know whether to eat or go right to sleep. This is a tough decision that athletes who finish late have to make on a regular basis. Keep in mind that your body does most of its repair work while you are sleeping, so if you find yourself in this situation try to come up with a solution in which you eat something light but are maximizing your sleep time. Just make sure that your solution doesn't involve fast food in any way.

Two hours after competition: This meal should be consumed when you are done competing for the day and THIS is where protein is the star of the show. At this point, you need protein to help rebuild all of the muscle that you broke down during competition. You also need lots of foods rich in chlorophyll to help restore alkalinity and speed recovery. Your post-competition meal should contain lots of leafy greens and antioxidants. Some people like to do a smoothie with a huge salad. That is a terrific option and I often do it myself. I would definitely advise against using a whey or casein protein in your smoothie. People are generally shocked when I say this, but most whey and casein supplements are milk by-products (not whole foods) and contribute to acidity as opposed to alkalinity. Soy protein isolate is really no better (depending on your unique food sensitivities, it might actually be worse). Whole food protein supplements made from rice, peas, hemp, and vegetables are much better sources of protein supplements, particularly post-competition. Quinoa is a complete protein and super-food that really shines as a post-workout meal. You can cook it with nuts, peas and spices to add extra protein and nutrient power.

I know that many of these principles are hard to apply at first. Eating a nutrient-dense diet is not really easy, especially if you travel a lot. When traveling with teams, I always bring a bag of my own super-foods, recovery mixes, and so on. You will get used to it as you should get used to reading labels and knowing what to avoid. All the effort is well worth it! You will recover faster and perform better on a consistent basis. You won't have those sluggish days when you can't figure out what went wrong. Trust me, that is worth a little extra planning.

CHAPTER SIX:
CAN VITAMIN WATER SEND YOU TO THE ER?

There is no air conditioning at the facility where I train my athletes. This has its advantages and disadvantages. One of the major advantages is that it is very similar to the heat and humidity that one might experience in game conditions. One of the disadvantages is that, pretty much every year, I get a girl who gets pretty close to passing out.

Luckily, I have only ever had one girl black out completely, and we took all of the necessary steps to make sure she was okay. I also made sure that they set up a doctor's appointment, just in case it wasn't the fact that she didn't eat or drink anything before her lesson that made her pass out.

As you can guess, it was the fact that she didn't eat or drink anything prior to her lesson that made her pass out. Also, did I mention she worked out before coming to her lesson?

Sooooo, let's try to avoid these kinds of situations shall we? Keep in mind that you always need to hydrate, but changes in altitude, humidity, air pressure and other variables can change your hydration needs.

One other thing that really affects hydration needs is how much caffeine you consume. You probably already know that caffeine is a diuretic. What that means is that it causes you to lose water through urination, which is not ideal if you are an athlete trying to hydrate to perform at an elite level. Caffeine is also a stimulant, so many of my athletes swear by having some coffee, tea, or (gasp!) soda (obviously I am not a proponent of this) before a game. There is even some research that suggests caffeine causes a short-term burst in performance.

But you must keep the following in mind: caffeine is not providing you with energy because it is giving you nutrients: it is providing you with energy because it is a stimulant. It will eventually wear off and leave you even more fatigued than you were to begin with. Caffeine is also taxing for the adrenal glands, resulting in production of the stress hormone cortisol. High levels of cortisol have been linked with inflammation, which is something you really want to minimize as an athlete.[42] High levels of cortisol have been linked to all sorts of other nasty things, including a decrease in the effectiveness of exercise and break down of muscle tissue. So if you are very dependent on coffee and other stimulants, try to cut back slowly. I cut out coffee all at once and got a massive headache for about three days. I stuck it out, but it wasn't particularly pleasant. I now get all my caffeine through tea (especially green tea and yerba mate), and if I have even a small amount of caffeinated coffee, I can't believe how insane and jittery I feel. That is not a good way to go through life! If you like the taste of coffee, try switching to decaffeinated. If you drink coffee only for the stimulation, gradually phase it out with some flavorful teas. You'll like the way you feel much better.

Can caffeine and stimulants actually be dangerous when it comes to hydration? I have a story for you.

---

[42]Brazier, Brendan. (2011). *Thrive Foods*. Cambridge, MA: Da Capo Press

I coached an athlete who currently plays Division I at a very competitive school. To know this girl and her family is to love them. They are incredibly hard workers, enthusiastic, and just as sweet as can be. Before she had signed her letter of intent, she was playing in a lot of showcases so that she could get recruited. On one such weekend, she was playing multiple games on a very hot day and drinking exclusively Vitamin Water. I am not a fan of Vitamin Water. Later that day, feeling very sick, she ended up in the emergency room with severe dehydration and heat exhaustion. How could this have happened if she was supposedly hydrating all day? You probably already guessed. The Vitamin water contained a stimulant that was also acting as a diuretic. She didn't feel thirsty since she felt like she was drinking, and that literally landed her in the emergency room. Thank God she recovered in a few days, but the whole situation should never have happened in the first place.

So that is why I am not a fan of any kind of Vitamin Water, since many of the formulations contain all different kinds of herbs and stimulants that might actually cause you to fail a NCAA drug test. You have to really be careful. I am also not a fan of Gatorade or Powerade since both are essentially just high fructose corn syrup. High fructose corn syrup has been shown to produce negative effects on metabolism and cause other problems and should therefore be avoided whenever possible.

So how can you stay hydrated? Here are some simple guidelines:

1. Drink 400 to 600 ml of water a half hour prior to activity. Since I work out in the morning, I always leave this amount of water next to my bedside and guzzle it first thing upon waking. This is not really my favorite thing to do, quite honestly, but I shoulder through it so I know I am hydrated for my workout. Everyone wakes up dehydrated (particularly if you are sunburned or if you had any alcoholic beverages the night before) because you haven't been able to drink anything for several hours. Drinking water first thing in the morning is a really

good habit to get into, particularly if you live in a warm climate.

2. Have lots of fluid during the early stages of practice and competition. You will absorb water better during this time.
3. Wear sunblock: I know that you all want to look tan, but sunblock is actually a coolant and will help to keep you from overheating (in addition to regular water consumption).
4. If you are sunburned, you are starting out a little dehydrated and will actually need more water than usual during competition.
5. Caffeine is a diuretic and can therefore dehydrate you. Stay away from beverages like Red Bull completely and watch out for drinks like Vitamin Water that can have herbs in them that are actually stimulants, even though the beverage is not labeled caffeinated.
6. If you are traveling by plane you are going to want to start drinking lots of water before you even get on the aircraft. There is no humidity on the inside of a plane and you will leave the plane feeling a little dehydrated if you don't drink plenty of fluids prior to getting on the plane and while you are on the plane. Be sure to drink the night before the plane trip as well.
7. Try to give yourself as much time as possible to acclimate to changes in humidity, altitude and so on if you are traveling to compete. You are a unique biological system that reacts differently to different climates and altitudes. If you are playing up in the mountains, altitude sickness is a real thing. Olympic athletes often arrive at the destinations where they are scheduled to compete a week (or longer) ahead of the competition. Gradually increase the intensity and duration of your training until you are acclimatized. You may need more to drink or more electrolytes than usual in a new environment.

So is water alone enough to hydrate you throughout your athletic activities?

It actually really depends. Water does not contain any electrolytes, and electrolytes are lost when you sweat. So if you are doing some light yoga or pilates, you probably aren't losing a lot of electrolytes unless you are a heavy sweater. If you are running a marathon, however, you will absolutely NEED electrolytes. So what are electrolytes? Electrolytes are minerals that carry an electrical charge. They have an impact on how your muscles function, how alkaline your blood is, and how much water you have in your body.

The following are electrolytes:

- Calcium
- Chloride
- Magnesium
- Phosphorous
- Potassium
- Sodium[43]

Here are some easy guidelines about consuming electrolytes:

1. You will need electrolytes more often than most athletes if you are a heavy sweater, or if you get white lines all over your clothing after you sweat. The appearance of white lines on your clothing after sweating indicates significant salt loss in your sweat.
2. If you are an average sweater, you will need electrolytes after an hour or more of activity.

Now comes the tricky part. What are the best ways to get electrolytes? Unfortunately, the problem with most electrolytes on the market is that they are largely composed of high fructose corn syrup, which has been shown to adversely affect metabolism and other functions of the body. I wouldn't drink anything with high fructose corn syrup. Ever. That stuff is pretty scary. Some people are starting to realize this and have become advocates of drinking coconut water instead. This makes quite a lot of sense, however, coconut water does not contain sodium. So unless you are adding salt to your coconut water, you are missing out on a very important electrolyte.

Making your own electrolyte drink is certainly a viable option, and there are many good recipes online that will allow you to do just that. It is actually pretty simple and certainly as natural as you can get. If you are like

[43] http://www.nlm.nih.gov/medlineplus/ency/article/002350.htm

me, though, I spend enough time doing food prep as it is without having to make my own electrolytes. So in my opinion, the powdered mixes are the way to go here. I like the Vega Brand Electrolyte Hydrator and also the Ultima brand. Both brands make tubs of electrolyte powders, but they also make (my favorite) little packets. Powders in general allow you to use more or less water to taste, which lets you adjust for your own preferences, but the great thing about the packets is that they are portable. I always leave an electrolyte packet in my purse and one in my sports bag in case I need it for any reason. It makes hydrating really simple since all you have to do is find water when you want to use it. There are so many times when I was thankful for keeping those little electrolyte packets with me. I use them frequently, but have also given them to my athletes on numerous occasions.

What if you feel like you simply cannot get enough electrolytes to perform properly? Maybe you just want to know the proportions of electrolytes in your urine and/or blood? Electrolytes can be tested in the laboratory by analyzing blood and/or urine. I have never known anyone who has had this test done, but it is available if you or your doctor think it is necessary.

One more note on electrolytes: it is possible to drink so much water that you dilute your electrolytes and suffer from low energy as a result. Keep this in mind if you have a tendency to drink a ton of water but never really take in electrolytes. It might make a huge difference in your energy levels and performance.

So what are the consequences of not hydrating properly? They can be very severe, actually. I have seen the affects firsthand and heard plenty of stories secondhand about the ill effects of even mild dehydration. Performance issues would be the least of your concerns if you are not properly hydrated. You might experience dizziness, nausea, vomiting, and other ill effects. The following are some things to look out for:

Heat exhaustion: It happens when there is not enough blood returning to the heart because the muscles and the skin are competing for blood. You will usually recognize the signs of heat exhaustion by the following:

-rapid, weak pulse

-low blood pressure

-faintness

-profuse sweating

-disorientation

If you or anyone on your team experiences this, you SHOULD NOT participate in any further activity for the rest of the day (at least). Here are some things that might help:

-Get an ice pack on specific trigger points

-Get to a cool area

-Drink plenty of water and electrolytes

-Rest

-My husband, who is a pharmacist, also recommends taking the athlete's temperature. Anything abnormally high should send you to the doctor ASAP.

Heat stroke: This is a major medical emergency. It means that the part of the brain that regulates temperature is no longer functioning as it should. Signs may sometimes vary, but the person typically becomes very confused or unconscious. This person should be kept as cool as possible (some sources suggest using ice) and taken to a hospital immediately.

I think that most people don't understand what a crucial role hydration plays in keeping us at peak performance (and keeping us alive!).

Follow the guidelines in this chapter and always take special precautions when adjusting to temperature changes. Most people are aware that they need to drink more when it is very hot, but you may not be as aware of your thirst if you are competing in the cold. You still need to drink! Test out your usage of water and electrolytes in your practices and training sessions to optimize your performance when game time rolls around.

CHAPTER SEVEN:
INJURY 911: RECOGNIZE AND PREVENT INJURIES

Most athletes are injured at some point in their careers. Injury that is a result of trauma is oftentimes completely unavoidable, but many injuries are a result of poor mechanics, overtraining, muscle fatigue and improper recovery methods. These are very preventable. Another problem that many athletes struggle with is distinguishing between muscular soreness and actual injury. This is understandable as the two can have similar characteristics. The goal of this chapter is to help you completely avoid preventable injuries, and help you to recognize when you are headed towards an injury as opposed to just experiencing soreness.

Have you noticed that you always get a cold (or worse) right at the peak of your training schedule? That is because overtraining can tax the immune system, muscles, and mind, making it more difficult for you to fight off infection. Training is important, but, contrary to popular belief, muscle growth does not occur when you are working out. It actually occurs during the rest phase. This happens because working out causes tiny tears in the muscles. The building of the muscles is essentially your body's adaptation to the stress. If you are constantly traumatizing the muscles, they will never get a chance to repair and grow. They will only ever break down. When constant break down is occurring, it leaves you in a weakened state where you are more susceptible to bad mechanics, injury, illness, and poor performance. As Brandon Marcello is fond of saying, "there is no such thing as overtraining, there is only under-recovering. "

Injuries can come in many different forms. Most people think of injuries starting with a specific trauma (i.e. sliding into third base and spraining an ankle), but many things can happen to make you susceptible to injury prior to the moment when you are actually hurt. For example, an outfielder might feel her shoulder give out on a throw to home. Though she suffers a severe injury in that throw, she was probably already experiencing tightness or imbalance in the shoulder that she ignored until the point of severe trauma.

Don't let this happen to you!

Here are some things that can contribute to a debilitating injury if left unchecked:

Fatigue: If you are playing intensely after a full night of studying or partying, you are much more likely to make mistakes and also more likely to be injured. After sixteen hours without sleep, attention, visual processing, decision-making and memory are all adversely affected. Twenty-two hours without sleep is the equivalent of having four shots of alcohol. Make sure that you are well-rested for both practices and games to make the most out of your athletic efforts.

Overuse: If you are hitting the same muscles continuously without rest and without any cross-training, those muscles are destined for injury. This type of training is also bound to eventually create muscular imbalances. Plan ahead each week to make sure you are mixing in strength training, balance, stretching and cardio. If you do not know which exercises work which muscles, spend time with a trainer or physical therapist to find out. This will help you to avoid constantly overworking certain areas while ignoring others. Great athletes are constantly pushing limits, and that is wonderful, but 6 days in a row of running is not serving anyone well. Rest or switch to an activity that requires use of different muscle groups on alternate days.

Tightness: It is never surprising to me when someone who has a tight lower back eventually pulls a hamstring. A tight lower back is usually one of the first signs that the hamstrings need attention, but many athletes ignore this sign until it is too late. Make a foam roller your best friend and use it for muscle prep prior to every strenuous activity. Since foam rollers don't necessarily travel well, I would also recommend purchasing a Tiger Tail muscle massager and a handball to work the tightness out of key areas of the body. Massage can also be a great tool to help alleviate tightness as long as you go to a licensed therapist. If you are constantly feeling tight no matter what you do, try to address the different stressors in your life that might make you feel that way. You would be surprised how much mental/emotional stress is related to inflammation and tightness.

Muscular Imbalance: Most athletes hit certain muscle groups much more frequently than others, thereby creating imbalance even when perfect mechanics are present. Avoid this problem by going for a Functional Movement Screening or having a physical therapist evaluate you. Twenty minutes of corrective exercise a day can improve your game and save you from injury.

Poor Nutrition: Eating poorly is one of the most common sources of inflammation and fatigue. If you don't give your body the tools it needs to fuel your workouts and help you to recover, then it cannot perform optimally. Period.

No Recovery Time/ Bad Recovery Methods: After a very intense workout or practice, you should actually be dedicating some time to recovery. This usually involves "cooling down" (i.e. getting the heart rate down), stretching, and then icing and doing a recovery snack within half an hour of the completed activity. Recovery can be much more involved if you have the time and the means or you are a professional athlete. If you are training for an Ironman triathlon for example, you should have a nap after your morning training. If you just ran ten miles, you might want to soak in a bath of Epsom salts. These are just some examples, but the muscles and mind will recover faster if you master recovery methods. You should also plan for resting muscle groups that you just worked intensely. So a pitcher who threw two hundred pitches on Saturday, even if she employs every great recovery technique, should not be throwing on Sunday. It is just too many reps in too short a period of time. It is particularly dangerous for young, developing bodies.

Incorrect Mechanics: Athletes need to understand the difference between a coach who will teach them a philosophy about how to move their bodies versus a coach who will look at each unique body structure and make appropriate adjustments based on biomechanics. For example, I often inherit young pitchers who twist their wrists into pretzels in an attempt to "get a better snap." There is simply no research whatsoever out there to support that this movement creates a better snap, but many coaches stand by it philosophically. This is a dangerous mindset that will not help you grow as an athlete. Find someone who knows what they are doing and can guide you through your career with minimal risk of injury.

Chronic Inflammation: Now, inflammation has a little bit of a bad rap, since it is actually one of the first adaptations your body makes in the recovery process. If you are constantly taking NSAIDS and anti-inflammatories, you actually may be increasing your recovery time and your risk of getting rebound headaches. Chronic inflammation on the other hand, is likely to lead to a lot of discomfort. Bad diet is a huge source of inflammation. That cheeseburger won't digest itself! Also, if you are always eating something that you may have sensitivity to, it is possible that it is increasing the levels of chronic inflammation in your body. Mental Stress (yes, you read that right), exhaustion, and overtraining can all contribute to chronic inflammation. Be kinesthetically aware, or keep a journal of how you feel during practices and training. This will allow you to know when to push your hardest, and when to back off a little.

Going From Zero to Sixty: People who take weeks off from their respective sport and then play four games in a weekend are pretty much asking to get injured. Many athletes make the mistake of throwing once or twice a week in preseason and then trying to increase to five/six times a week in season. This is a recipe for disaster. Track your pitch count every time you practice and know how many pitches you can throw before you start to fatigue and compromise your mechanics. If you are a distance runner, you should be gradually increasing your mileage and then tapering. You wouldn't prepare to run a 5K and then run a marathon. Other athletes should think of training in the same way. Remember that if you build up too quickly without scheduling rest and recovery, your body will force you to rest, generally in the form of an illness or injury.

No matter what your sport, there are some things you should do prior to engaging in activity that can lessen your chances of injury and enhance your performance. Foam rolling or any sort of muscle rolling is the best way to start out since it loosens the tissue and generally increases mobility. Warming up is something that every athlete should execute on every plane of motion. Going for a jog is not necessarily a great warm up because it only works the muscles in the sagittal plane (the front of the body). Sports don't only happen on one plane of motion. You want to make sure that you do dynamic movements in the frontal plane (like sliding sideways) and transverse plane (going across the body) as well as the sagittal plane, since this more accurately reflects how you will move in your workouts. Static stretching (stretching while standing still) is typically not great before a workout, although dynamic stretching (stretching through engaging in different movements on different planes) is fine. Static stretching is typically best used after the workout or competition. I find the following to be the best way to warm up pre-competition: foam roll, do a dynamic warm up, and activate your muscles. This should leave you ready to work out intensely.

Following an intense activity, you should do a cool down (getting your heart rate down). For runners, this may be as simple as walking for a bit after a race. Pitchers might want to do a quick version of their warm-up backwards. After the cool down phase, static stretching should follow every competition, training session and workout. Yes, you should stretch AFTER you play. Why? Your muscles shorten after the constant contraction of playing. If you don't stretch them afterwards, they become tight and potentially imbalanced. This problem then becomes worse if the next thing you do is sit on a bus to travel for 4 hours. Remember that tightness and imbalance are 2 things that contribute to injuries. You will reap tremendous benefits from just a little extra time at the end of your workouts. Cooling down and stretching also give you time to reflect on the game or workout and determine what you can do to better yourself as an athlete.

Let's assume you have been following all the guidelines I have given you thus far. You have been practicing hard: throwing seemingly endless hours every week to perfect your motion. You are doing weight training and cardio to help you cross-train. You have been warming up, cooling down and stretching. Despite all of this, you are definitely feeling some discomfort. What to do?

The problem is that if you stop training every time you are a little sore or have a case of the sniffles, you will probably never get in enough hours of quality practice to meet your ultimate goals. So if you are sore after some high-intensity exercise, low-intensity exercise the following day can actually help to reduce soreness. Train at 30-40 % of the effort you expended in your high-intensity workout and see how you feel the next day.[44]

---

[44] http://www.drmikemarshall.com/TheScienceofEnergyExpenditure.html

On the other hand, if you keep practicing and training while you are hurt, you will only make things worse. Here are some signs that you might be injured (as opposed to just sore), so it might be time to back off a little and/or see a professional:

You have visible swelling: This is pretty self-explanatory, but if your forearm is hurting and is visibly larger than usual, you better take a day or two off. You also need to determine what the cause of the inflammation is. Oftentimes, I will see a pitcher at my facility complaining of discomfort in her elbow or forearm. Generally, my first question is, "are you hitting your hip?" Most girls will quickly respond, "no." A quick glimpse at the area around the elbow will tell us if they are mistaken. If there is visible swelling around the area of the elbow due to the repeated trauma of hitting the hip, we know that is the culprit. If this is left unchecked, it will definitely cause an injury.

The area of discomfort is hot to the touch: This is generally indicative of a high level of inflammation and you should not be practicing when the tissue is inflamed to this degree.

You lost range of motion: If you have worked out so excessively that you cannot lift your arms over your head the next day, there is no way that you should be working out that area again. If you have consistently decreased range of motion over a period of weeks, it's time to get it checked out.

The area in question is unstable: Instability can potentially be a sign that there is a tear. Just to be clear, this is not the same as having bad balance, since balance is an area that most athletes need to improve. I am referring to the type of instability that occurs when you feel something "give out." For example, if you have discomfort in your knee, particularly from doing a violent motion or a change in direction, you might feel a little better after the initial trauma. However, if you walk down the stairs leading with that leg that and that knee gives out on you, you should absolutely get it checked. That can be a sign of an ACL or meniscal tear. Similarly, if your shoulder is bothersome, and you can't hold a yoga plank position without it giving out, you need to get it checked.

You are unable to "loosen up": Sometimes, you are just a little stiff or sore and need to work through some of the discomfort by moving slowly and deliberately initially. This is naturally going to happen when you are trying to push yourself to the limit. When you are sore in this way, heat and foam rolling are an amazing combination to use prior to your workout. If things loosen up after heat and foam rolling, you are probably okay to do a light workout. If, however, you cannot get the offending area to loosen up after taking the aforementioned steps, you should definitely rest that day. Monitor the area the following day(s).

The soreness is continually coming back to the same area: This doesn't necessarily mean that you are injured, although it is a possibility. Soreness can sometimes just be a sign of working new muscles. For example, if you have never used your legs in your pitch before, when you first use them to their full potential, the legs will be sore again and again while the muscle is building. In other instances, however, soreness that is repeatedly showing up in the same area can be a sign that you are either throwing with incorrect mechanics, overtraining, or perhaps have a fracture or some connective tissue damage. I did once have an athlete who had a "sore finger" for several weeks, and it turned out that it was actually broken. Tough girl. You wouldn't want to face her in a fight. As tough as she is though, not knowing that her finger was broken cost her weeks of recovery. It is always better to be cautious. If you feel that your soreness could possibly be a result of incorrect mechanics, go to someone who specializes in biomechanics or have a physical therapist watch your motion. I made the mistake of pitching with torn cartilage in my wrist for over a year because I spent a long time writing it off as soreness or tendinitis. That cost me a lot of time. It cost hours and hours of training, recovery, and development. I spent over a year not throwing or training to my full potential when I should have been addressing the problem. Don't let this happen to you! That year is my biggest regret as an athlete and I want to help other athletes avoid this mistake.

The pain is sharp and/or shooting: There are only very rare instances in which shooting pain is NOT a cause for concern. I would suggest taking the day off and getting this checked immediately if I were you.

Remember, there is no possible way to avoid every single potential injury, but following the guidelines laid out in this chapter should help you to avoid most. They should also help you to seek the proper help and rest when these things are necessary. I am extremely passionate about helping athletes to avoid injury since I lost so much time to injury myself.

CHAPTER EIGHT:
RECOVER LIKE A SUPERHERO

Unfortunately, we sometimes get injured despite our best efforts to avoid it. When this happens, we are usually desperate to get back to activity. The idea of having to take a few weeks off is generally awful to a competitive athlete. So I am providing you with some resources to help you get back in the game quickly after a soft tissue injury and help you learn the art of recovery after a strenuous workout. As you read this, though, do remember that caution is always very important when it comes to returning to full activity after an injury. Many athletes want to play so badly that they risk playing on a sprained ankle (or worse) and, in doing so, compromise both their health and their mechanics. This is only going to hurt your performance in the long run.

If you are injured or have been injured in the past, see if this scenario sounds familiar:

1. You have pain
2. You got to see your primary care doctor
3. Your doctor orders x-rays
4. The x-rays show nothing and the pain gets worse
5. Your primary care decides to refer you to a specialist
6. The specialist orders a battery of tests
7. Three weeks have gone by and you have gotten nowhere

This is a very common scenario. The issue is that your primary care is not an orthopedist or physiatrist, nor does she have the resources that a physical therapist does, where you can be started on corrective exercises right away. I am certainly NOT saying that you should avoid a trip to your primary care, it is always good for them to know about any health issues you have, but you should probably be doing a few other things at the same time.

Personally, if I feel that I have some kind of soft tissue injury, my first stop is actually to my physical therapist. Why? My physical therapist happens to be one of the best diagnosticians I have ever met (and I am picky picky picky). If he is not sure what is causing the problem, he has a network of people whom he trusts that he will refer me to. This saves me A LOT of wasteful doctor's visits, especially since my insurance is pretty basic (read: crappy), to put it mildly. Seeing my awesome physical therapist also gets me back in the game faster, since he will give me exercises that very day to do at home. He usually also prescribes me a regimen of heat, ice, or stretching. I can literally start getting better the same day that I go to visit him. So, basically, make sure that you develop a good relationship with an expert physical therapist in your area specializing in working with athletes (preferably in your sport). I once went to a physical therapy office that apparently specialized in treating older individuals, and it is quite a different scenario. They use different modalities and have different areas of expertise. Do your homework on the best sports physical therapists in your area, and if there aren't any in your area, trust me, it is worth it to travel a bit.

Something that many people do not know is that physical therapists can often see you for one visit before you need to get a referral from an MD, depending on your insurance. The physical therapist might even be able to help you to find the best MD possible for your condition. If you are lucky, the physical therapist might only need to see you once before diagnosing a problem that they commonly see. Remember that primary care doctors often have more experience in infections, vaccinations, blood work, and so forth. They may only see a few sports injuries in a week, whereas a physical therapist sees sports injuries countless times a day. I have also noticed that all good physical therapists will request that you perform your athletic motion for them (whether you are a hockey player, pitcher, runner, etc.). This way, they can correct mechanical things that might be compromising your joints, ligaments, tendons and so forth. The physical therapist might even be able to get you on a fast track to recovery because he is already familiarized with your specific sport and your specific injury. He is also better equipped than an MD to address your questions about stretching, heating versus icing, and general recovery times for injury.

Different physical therapists use different modalities to help improve your condition. You might be introduced to ultrasound, electric stimulation, and even laser treatment. Some therapists might also want to use hydrocortisone cream or suggest a cortisone injection. The thing that you must remember before subjecting yourself to a cortisone injection is that it will NOT actually heal the damaged tissue. In fact, studies show that it may even make the area more likely to rupture in the future. Cortisone is really more for pain management, but pain does tell you when you should stop! Do your homework if you are considering a cortisone shot, and consider some of the alternative therapies mentioned later in this chapter.

Once such alternative therapy is called ART (short for Active Release Technique). This is a great resource if you are suffering from a soft tissue injury. Professional and Olympic athletes expedite healing of soft tissue injuries by using ART. ART helps to break up the scar tissue caused by soft tissue damage and helps increase blood flow and range of motion in an injured area. I will warn you that it is NOT a comfortable process, but it is highly useful. I pulled an intercostal muscle (rib muscle) a while back. It is a notoriously difficult problem to address. A pulled intercostal is very painful and usually lasts a long time. I was about 90 percent better with only two ART treatments. I was back to normal workouts in no time. If you go to a responsible provider, this technique really works. ART is a modality that many physical therapists use, but you don't need to be in physical therapy to reap the benefits. Many chiropractors and massage therapists are also certified. You can go to their website at www.ActiveRelease.com to find a provider near you. I would even recommend going if you are constantly tight in one area since, as you may recall, muscular tightness and imbalance can create injury in the long run.

KT tape and/or Kinesio tape are two other great resources for soft tissue damage. The major difference between the two is that Kinesio tape is generally applied by certified Health Care providers, while KT tape can be bought at a sporting goods store and applied according to directions on their website: www.kttape.com. These tapes work by promoting circulation to the area, supporting the joints, and generally promoting the body's natural healing processes. Kinesio tape is better if you have a somewhat unusual injury, or one that is not addressed on the KT tape website. Health care providers who do Kinesio taping have hours and hours of experience and can often tape almost any soft tissue injury to help alleviate discomfort. Many physical therapists are also certified in Kinesio taping, but other healthcare providers are as well. If you can't find someone who does Kinesio taping in your area, or you decide to use KT tape on your own, YOU MUST follow directions. I certainly don't recommend just buying tape and slapping it all over your body willy nilly. According to my physical therapist, this is actually more common than you might think. If it is not applied correctly, you will not be reaping the benefits of this modality. Use the resources on the website or leave it to the professionals.

Some physical therapists also use massage therapy, but you can also go to a licensed massage therapist (again, someone who specializes in sports is preferable!). This is a great resource when you are injured or even if you are just tight or stressed. Just be sure to ask your physical therapist or orthopedist if massage is appropriate for your specific injury since, in some cases, massage might not be appropriate. In patellar tendinitis, for example, massage might actually aggravate the injury. In general, I like to tell my athletes to go for a massage when they have tightness that is always returning to one area of the body. Massage is also good if they have completely overworked themselves and need a little help healing from that overworked state. Massage is a great tool for preventing injury when utilized properly, but is also generally good for the lymphatic system.

Recent research from the University of Illinois concluded that massage administered after working a group of sedentary adults to fatigue found improved blood flow for 48 hours after the massage. The group that received the massage also did not experience soreness as compared with the control group. The control group experienced soreness for 24 hours.[45] A recent study in The International Journal of Sports Physical Therapy also showed promising results for self-massage (i.e. work with a foam roller) after a strenuous workout (45). This is definitely a method of recovery to look into! Just make sure that you drink plenty of water prior to your massage and throughout the day afterwards.

Though I have not been treated with Muscle Activation Technique myself, many people have raved about its effectiveness. I took a day-long course on the basics of MAT several years ago and thought the principles were very sound. What little I know of MAT has been effective with my athletes when other techniques have not worked. I would love to have done the full certification, but I need the time! The concept behind MAT is that inefficient muscle contractions lead to decreased range of motion and physical performance. These inefficient muscle contractions can also manifest as pain. An MAT practitioner will evaluate your ability to perform efficient muscle contractions and then apply forces to help the deficient muscle(s) contract correctly. You can get more information at http://www.muscleactivation.com.

Another little-known option for athletes who are experiencing pain is to seek a physiatrist. A physiatrist is a medical doctor who specializes in rehabilitation and generally works with a team of professionals to help the athlete recover without surgery. Physiatrists do an initial evaluation, and then, based on that evaluation, they try to develop a program for helping

---

[45] (2014 July-August). Latest Research on Massage and Exercise-Induced Muscle Soreness. IDEA Fitness Journal, 11(7), 11.

the client to heal and stay active. They often work closely with physical therapists. Since physiatrists are MDs, however, they do have the ability to write prescriptions and may suggest a course of either oral or topical anti-inflammatories or NSAIDS. Cortisone shots are a very common way that orthopedists and other medical doctors address inflammation, but remember that there is mounting evidence to support the theory that these shots can actually weaken the structure and make it more likely to rupture down the road. If you are opposed to this kind of treatment, voice your concerns to the doctor.

Many people have already been to chiropractors, but they are still considered "alternative medicine" for the most part. I have been to several different chiropractors in my life and have only ever had a bad experience with one (whom I never went back to). If the pain that you have is resulting from something that is structural, (for example you have a misalignment in your thoracic spine), an adjustment from a chiropractor specializing in treating athletes can make you feel better a lot faster. Make sure you get the name of a knowledgeable chiropractor from someone you trust and someone who has been treated by him. You should also know that there are at least two different kinds of chiropractors. There are upper cervical chiropractors and general chiropractors. I think that both are good, so do your homework before deciding which kind is right for you. Both types of chiropractors believe that misalignments interrupt the communications of the nerve system. Upper cervical chiropractors believe that the disruption occurs in an area called the atlas, which is at the very top of your spine. Most upper cervical chiropractors will write a script for you to get very specific x-rays taken before they will treat you. They typically use an instrument during every visit to determine whether or not the atlas is properly aligned. This means that if you go to see an upper cervical chiropractor, you will not get adjusted at every single visit. You will only be adjusted when the scan is off. Many general chiropractors also use instruments to measure a client. General chiropractors will sometimes use things like scanners or machines that check temperature, but they mostly do not use these things every visit. They often check the client through palpation (feel) instead. Upper cervical chiropractors will adjust you while you are in a kneeling position, whereas general chiropractors will mostly adjust you while you are lying or your back or your side.[46] [47]

When I had stopped tennis a while ago because of some back pain, the owner of a local tennis facility had referred me to an acupuncturist. I was a little skeptical and kind of frightened at first. I don't like needles and I really didn't know much about acupuncture. Fortunately, I decided to give it a try. I am so thankful that I did! My acupuncturist is kind, incredibly intelligent, hilarious, and so knowledgeable of all different kinds of natural remedies. I pretty much use him as most people would use a primary care: "I've had two colds in a month, what do I do?" He is always there with a smile and a very good answer. Acupuncture has been the subject of much research as of late, and even Western trained doctors are acknowledging its effectiveness. The needles are tiny. It is not always comfortable while it is happening, but you feel amazing afterwards. Don't just look up any random acupuncturist online. Find someone you can build a relationship with and trust. There are many acupuncturists near my house, but I travel a half hour out of my way to see mine. Don't ever compromise your health for convenience.

Ayurvedic Medicine is another alternative therapy that most people know very little about. For those of you already familiar with the research showing that turmeric and boswellia (or frankincense) are both effective in treating inflammatory conditions, you can thank Ayurveda. Ayurveda is one of the oldest medical systems. It originated in India over 3,000 years ago. Practitioners of Ayurveda evaluate the body's constitution, life forces (dosha) and the state of interconnectedness to create unique treatments for patients. These treatments often include herbs, massage, and/or diet and lifestyle changes. There have not been many formal studies on the

---

[46] http://atlas4wellness.com/uc%20vs%20chiro.htm

[47] http://www.sciencebasedmedicine.org/the-problem-with-chiropractic-nucca/

effectiveness of Ayurvedic medicine, but there are some good documentaries that explore its uses. I have also heard stories of people who have solved ongoing problems by using this modality. You must be careful if you are prescribed herbs from any health care practitioner, however, since some herbs can interact with conventional medications or be dangerous if not dosed correctly. You must also remember that herbs and supplements are, as of right now, not regulated at all, so pretty much anything can be in them. Always read labels and, if you are inclined to try any kind of herbal remedy, try to find one that is organically sourced and made in the USA, since some of the herbs and other products from overseas have been shown to contain metals and toxins. Always make sure that all of your healthcare providers know what you are taking. I went to a short seminar on Ayurveda several years ago, but have never been to see a practitioner. I think, like anything, the most important thing is the quality of the person whom you go to for treatment. Since Ayurveda is not commonly practiced in the United States, it might be hard to find someone with good qualifications, so as always, do your homework.[48]

Orthotics are a tool that have really fallen out of favor now that the barefoot running movement is in vogue. I have been to seminars on barefoot running and have also heard from the side arguing for orthotics. The problem with barefoot running is that you have been using shoes your entire life and suddenly trying to run long distances without support can leave you susceptible to stress fractures. I think the idea of running for a minute a day barefoot on a soft surface is a reasonable idea and will probably help to strengthen some of the muscles in the feet that are infrequently used. As a long-term practice over long distances, however, barefoot running could potentially be dangerous. Your body does move

[48] http://nccam.nih.gov/health/ayurveda/introduction.htm

from the ground up, so if there is an existing problem such as severe pronation, supination, or a change in the structure of your foot as a result of the movements your sport requires (hello to my pitchers), orthotics might be really helpful. Some people who make orthotics will simply have you step into a mold and make an insert from that. I had that done many years ago (before becoming vegan) after tearing my posterior tibial tendon. I don't think this is the best way to go. I have since had orthotics made with someone who took very specific measurements and spent a lot of time asking me questions and changing my foot position. He was a physical therapist who chose to specialize in orthotics. This is the way to go. Any professional who really spends this kind of time with you and is willing to make adjustments to the final product to suit your needs is going to just be better overall.

There are some things that you can use at home if you are injured or sore. Soaking in a bath of Epsom salts (follow the directions on the package) can be very soothing. It helps draw stored tissue wastes, and therefore inflammation, from the body. As Dr. Hanes said, "Epsom salts contain all-natural magnesium, which helps your muscles relax and stop aching" (April 2014 issue of *Health*). Currently there are even "floatation centers" that allow clients to float in a room where there is essentially a pool filled with Epsom salts. These centers boast that floatation practice is good for everything from muscle recovery to reducing stress hormones and aiding the immune system. This is because magnesium sulfate is absorbed through the skin while you are soaking in the bath.

As far as over-the-counter pain relief is concerned, arnica is a very useful topical treatment for aiding in healing bruises and easing joint and muscle pains. Just make sure you are not allergic and that it is okay with your health care provider. Arnica is very effective but, like any medication, it can be dangerous in very large doses.

Walk into any natural foods store and ask for something to take orally that will help with inflammation. Let me guess: they suggested that you take either some form of cumin or turmeric. Psychic! So are cumin and turmeric safe? They are both spices! If you have an adventurous and worldly pantry like mine, you can actually find those little anti-inflammatory gems right in there. As you already know, I am not a big believer in taking lots of pills, so I like to include these spices in the foods that I eat as much as possible. If you eat a lot of Indian food, you are probably already getting lots of both spices. If you are feeling like you need a little more concentrated form of these spices to speed up the recovery process, however, these are both pretty safe as long as you are healthy and have no allergies to either. Always check with your health care provider to avoid contraindications with other medications or herbs, and ALWAYS check to make sure the ingredients are organic and have no weird fillers or other additives.

All athletes should have access to heating pads and ice packs. Heat is generally used before activity to help promote blood flow, while ice is used after to decrease inflammation, but many health care practitioners have been promoting going back and forth between hot and cold: a method known as "pumping." Since some injuries benefit more from ice, and others from heat, it is always good to check with your PT regarding your specific injury.

Sleep is one of the best ways for your body to recover, so you must take this aspect of your training very seriously. Try to schedule eight hours. Make sure that there is no use of electronic devices before you go to sleep at night and keep the room you sleep in as dark as possible. Don't have any sugar or alcohol before you go to bed as these things (as well as light) all disrupt the sleep cycle and prevent you from recovering optimally. Also try not to have any large meals before bed. If you think that sleep isn't all that important, do your homework. Amazing athletes in all sports from LeBron James to Michelle Wie and Rafael Nadal swear by getting *at least* 8 hours a night.

Finally, for optimal recovery, eat lots of leafy green vegetables and fruits. The chlorophyll and antioxidants will help promote cell recovery.

Remember, once you have been injured, you can easily reinjure that area if your mechanics are not what they should be or if you try to return to activity too quickly. Make sure you have someone evaluating your sports motion. If you have had multiple soft tissue injuries with the same instructor, the hard truth is that you should probably look for someone new. Your current instructor might not be addressing the root of the problem. Also, work on becoming more kinesthetically aware. Once you know your body better (i.e. understanding soreness versus strain versus exhaustion) you will be better able to prevent injuries and recover from them.

CHAPTER NINE:
CONQUERING CROSS-TRAINING CHALLENGES

Athletes typically don't understand much about cross-training. Though the right cross-training can really enhance performance, simply throwing around some weights at the gym in addition to your normal training and practice might actually decrease your performance if you (or your trainer) don't know what you are doing. It is therefore really important to understand the difference between training ideologies, corrective movement analysis, "prehab," and trainers who are just out to make money.

There are some things that all good cross-training programs have in common:

1. They treat the body globally. In other words, they don't just train one specific area or muscle group, but try to make all of the muscles work together harmoniously. If you have been tested for certain weaknesses or imbalances you might have to do some work in isolation, but most of your training should be global.

2. They work on different planes of movement. There are three planes of motion: transverse, frontal and sagittal plane. Some complementary training programs have you work on just one plane of motion standing still. This is not generally how sports or life happen. You have to change direction, sometimes very quickly, and your training should accommodate for that.

111

3. They teach you how to accelerate and decelerate properly. These are the movements that athletes are most frequently injured doing, so it is important to understand how they work.

4. They should incorporate range of motion and flexibility. If you are really strong, but not flexible at all, that will eventually be a hindrance for you. It can leave you more susceptible to injury or simply prevent you from being able to execute an athletic movement efficiently.

5. They should address the mental aspect of training. Once your mechanics are pretty good and you reach a higher level, most of your success or failure will have to do with mental preparation (which we will discuss in later chapters). Though you might want to do some work with a therapist if you are having major issues with confidence or anxiety, there are things you can do on your own. A good cross-training program will help you learn to focus, push hard, and thrive in competition.

6. They should address balance. All sports involve balance. Anyone who tells you otherwise is misinformed. Working on balance doesn't mean standing on your head on a bosu ball or performing circus tricks. What it does involve is focus and the activation of lots of different muscles in the kinetic chain. Yoga is perfect for this type of work.

7. They should have at least one part of the workout where you are learning to push to your limits. As someone who takes your sport very seriously, you need to know how hard you can actually push yourself. Sometimes I am shocked at what my body can do and sometimes I am aggravated by what it can't. If you are always doing a workout that is easy for you or doesn't challenge you mentally, then there is no way you will be able to stand up to the challenges presented on game/race day.

8. They should leave appropriate time for recovery. There are some people who think it is okay to go to Crossfit everyday. This is just nuts. If you are pushing your limits every time you go to training, you have to take at least a day of rest (or yoga) in between and start incorporating some good recovery habits (see "Recover Like a Superhero").

Probably the best place to start with complementary training is "prehab." The idea behind prehab is to prevent an injury before it starts. This process begins by getting evaluated by a physical therapist or athletic trainer. Based on the results of the evaluation, you are prescribed corrective exercises and stretches. Your prehab program should hopefully address any deficiencies and/or imbalances. This is something that I would recommend for serious athletes of all ages. You will have a customized workout program designed to keep you at your best on the court, track, or field.

Similarly, many healthcare professionals offer what is called a Functional Movement Screening. Developed by a physical therapist, this program is comprehensive and very useful. You go through a series of tests when you are screened, which check for flexibility, range of motion, and form. Based on the results, you and your health care professional create a personalized account on the FMS website. You log in and your exercises are posted daily with descriptions, pictures, and occasionally video. These are tools designed to help you execute the movements properly. The exercises are posted in such a way that they increase in difficulty over time, so you have to make sure that you do them consistently. After several weeks, you get evaluated again and are typically given different exercises based on the improvements you made since the first screening. FMS is a very good program, with only one disadvantage: it is sometimes hard to determine whether or not you are doing the exercises correctly. I would suggest asking the person who evaluates you to watch you do the first set of exercises in your account. In this way, you will ensure that you are going through the movements correctly and therefore receiving the benefits of all of your extra work.

Every single athlete, regardless of sport, should be doing yoga as complementary training. Study after study demonstrates the benefits of mind/body training. Yoga improves flexibility, concentration, balance, and focus, among other things. There are many different styles of yoga, so you can find one that resonates with you. For me, hatha yoga is pretty much perfect, but definitely go out and explore. I do not recommend "hot yoga" at all, however. The temperatures can be dangerously hot, leaving you at risk for dehydration and heat exhaustion. Additionally, the intense heat warms your muscles, so you are under the false impression that you can stretch further than you are actually capable of stretching. Along with yoga comes meditation, which is so important for stilling the mind, especially since, as an athlete, you've got a lot going on up there (more on meditation in later chapters).

For those of you interested in exploring Pilates or Tai Chi, these are also great forms of complementary training that incorporate a mind-body connection. Make sure that you choose at least one discipline that will allow you to "zone in" and find the right balance between being engaged and relaxed, since this is an integral part of success in sports at a higher level.

One very important component of complementary training is the idea that, if you are very young, most of your cross-training should come from playing other sports. I hate hearing about 9 and 10 year-olds already specializing in one sport or another and giving up everything else. This means that those young athletes are taxing the same muscles and joints over and over again without any reprieve. This is especially true now that almost all sports can be played year-round. Additionally, a dangerous trend I have noticed over the last several years is the tendency towards making sports for athletes ages 10 and under highly competitive. That is borderline insane. At 10 and under, athletes should be receiving instruction, and not getting screamed at if they bobble a ball. Research shows that very young athletes benefit the most simply from engaging in activities like running, jumping, crawling, swimming, and so forth. Creating early specialization is pretty much an overuse injury and/or burnout waiting to happen.

Since I opened the book discussing Crossfit, everyone probably assumes that I think it is great for complementary training. The truth is, I have very mixed feelings about that, depending on your sport and your level of competitiveness. If the people who own your gym have integrity, force you do to the movements correctly, and don't have you go up in weight too quickly, then I think CrossFit can be decent OFF-SEASON training for some sports. Notice the emphasis on "off-season." Doing Crossfit in the same season as your primary sport would be very much like playing two sports in the same season and is definitely not advisable. If you are the type of athlete who only works hard when you have heavy competition, Crossfit might be a good match for you. For me, it has been eye-opening how hard I can actually push myself. There are also so many different movements to learn in Crossfit, it can be tough to keep track and master all of them. You definitely need to keep a notebook, watch lots of videos on proper form, and talk to your instructors about how well you are executing technique. If your Crossfit instructors don't seem to care, you are at a bad gym and should leave immediately. At the Crossfit I go to, they won't let us do certain movements until we master others, hence there is constant modification and the instructors have integrity and are on top of everyone. There is also a great sense of community (very much like a team) that makes everyone encourage everyone else. In one instance, I can remember a new member of our Crossfit taking so long to finish his workout that he overlapped into the next class. It didn't matter, though, since everyone in the next class was cheering him on and congratulating him when he finally finished. He felt great and felt supported. That's tough to get at a regular gym.

One of the main problems with Crossfit, however, is the constant emphasis on going heavier and heavier. Increasing your weight a lot over a very short period of time is typically a very good recipe for getting hurt. On the other hand, you should challenge yourself somewhat. This is where a very clever trainer has come up with the idea of using biofeedback to help clients determine when to safely increase their weight. Biofeedback is a technique in which clients are connected to electrical sensors to help them receive information about their bodies. These sensors "send signals to a monitor, which displays a sound, flash of light, or image that represents your heart and breathing rate, blood pressure, skin temperature, sweating, or muscle activity."[49] Having this information allows you to become more aware of changes in your body and it allows you to relax or activate certain muscles. As you use the images on the screen to slow your heart rate, lower

---

[49] http://www.webmd.com/a-to-z-guides/biofeedback-therapy-uses-benefits

your blood pressure, and lessen the tightness in your muscles, you'll get instant feedback on the screen. Eventually, you will learn how to control these functions on your own, without the screen. Biofeedback is also used to help alleviate stress, headaches, and chronic pain.

I recently read some idiot's blog saying that softball players don't need to cross-train with any cardio. The fact that information like that is even read by anyone pretty much just makes me see red. All athletes, regardless of sport, should be doing some sort of appropriate cardio for cross-training. I do understand the arguments against long-distance running or long-distance biking as forms of cardio since long-distance running can be rough on the joints and back. Long-distance biking is definitely not an ideal posture to be in. Additionally, these movements only happen on one plane of movement (the sagittal plane), and sports happen in many different planes of motion (the frontal plane, the sagittal plane and the transverse plane). Swimming can be good cardio and it avoids pounding on the joints. There are so many different swimming strokes that you can easily work on different planes of motion. Rowing and jump rope can also be good cardio, but probably the best cardio I have seen so far was at Stanford when I shadowed Brandon Marcello for a week. He does something with the athletes called "Energy Systems Development," which is apparently a euphemism for brutal cardio interspersed with periods of rest. He had them doing many different exercises on many different planes of motion at different stations. They would go as hard as they could 12 seconds and then take 24 seconds to recover. They did this for an hour.

Bodybuilding is definitely a sport, but it is not a good tool for cross-training. Body-building creates beautiful muscle, but that muscle might not be functional for your particular sport. It might even over-develop certain muscle groups or decrease flexibility: two things that can actually hurt your performance. Many personal trainers out there are body-builders and train their clients that way. Remember, not all personal trainers and athletic trainers are created equally. Always try to look for someone who specializes in your sport and has a history of helping athletes *in your sport* get to the next level without hurting them.

TRX training and the Jungle Gym are two very similar types of complementary training. In both systems, straps are attached to a bar or tucked into a door. The athlete then uses the straps for various exercises. Most of these exercises involve balancing to some degree as well as training the muscles. The TRX or Jungle Gym can provide a terrific total body workout when used properly. Athletes can do leg work by putting one foot in the straps or by gripping the straps for some support with pistols (one-legged squats). There are so many different upper body exercises that can be done on these devices and you can actually do some pretty difficult abdominal exercises as well. Just always do your homework before getting started. Many gyms have started TRX classes and the Jungle Gym comes with a DVD.

What I have noticed as a trend over the last several years is that many teams will do some sort of cross-training program over the winter. This very often involves going to a "training facility" (notice the quotes) once a week or even once every two weeks where a "trainer" has them do very advanced compound exercises or exercises they are not yet strong enough to do. The athletes are usually sore for several days after and, obviously, if you are only doing cross-training once a week, you are not getting anything out of it. Particularly with young athletes, it is essential that they learn how to do basic training movements before they move onto anything as advanced as compound exercises. They should never be so sore from training that they can't move the next day. In general, unless you have someone really familiar with your sport working with your team or making accommodations for different player positions and/or differences in strength and anatomy, you are probably better off doing cross-training on your own. In all my years as a personal trainer and coach, I have never once seen an athlete make gains from the aforementioned types of training. I have only seen them get exhausted and hurt.

Balance training was incredibly popular several years ago and is definitely still used in most training facilities. Balance training typically includes a bosu ball (that thing that looks like a half ball), a stability ball (the big ball that you can lie on) or, sometimes, small pods. Though I do think stability training is effective in small doses, you should definitely be starting with yoga if your balance is not great. Lifting dumbbells on top of a Bosu ball is really just silly. Additionally, throwing yourself right into balance training without any prior training is going to increase your chance of injury.

So now you are probably thinking, "but I can't do anything with fancy equipment for cross-training and I don't have a gym membership. What about those P90X videos or Jillian Michaels videos?" First of all, let me preface this by saying that Jillian Michaels is a friend in my head. Meaning, I have never met her, but I think we are oddly alike and I find her entertaining and engaging. I know some personal trainers hate her, and I totally don't get that. Don't be hating on Jillian, she does some good things! I do own quite a few of her videos. I think her "Yoga Meltdown" video is a great way to train. It makes Yoga into a cardio sweatfest, which is really fun. On the flip side, the kettle bell video ("Shred it with Weights"), while fun, does not really utilize good kettle bell form, so I would stay away from that one. Also, some of her videos go directly into complicated moves really quickly, and if you are new to working out, it might be a little too complicated. Use caution with any video systems, because, of course, there is no one there to spot you and make sure that you are doing it correctly.

Tony Horton's P90X is also really fun, but some of the exercises are awkward (push-ups with hands set up unevenly) and there are also lots of compound exercises, so again, bad idea for beginners and young athletes. I also found that P90X made me really really tight (more so than Crossfit) and I subsequently pulled a muscle. That might just be my individual experience, but approach with caution. Do yourself a favor if you plan on doing any video workouts and watch the workout at least once first. Use good judgment. If the moves depicted in the video are overcomplicated, awkward, or beyond your current level of fitness, stick to something simpler. Your library is an amazing resource for fitness DVDs. That is how I have done sooo many different ones. I have done everything from

Zumba to P90X and back again (incidentally, Zumba is really fun but probably not the best cross-training). You can try these videos out and then return them. If you're lucky, your library might even carry a sports-specific DVD (like "Training for Tennis," or something similar).

Finally, a unique idea for training is integrating different cross-training movements into your athletic motion. For example, I often have my pitchers try to throw on one leg for balance (we playfully call this "pitching yoga") or try to throw in a plank position to work on core stability. This is one of those things that doesn't look really impressive until you try it (for some examples, go to www.flawlessfastpitch.com). You can integrate speed work by doing your athletic motion with light resistance (typically using bands or bungees) or by doing your motion (generally without the ball) slowly in a pool. The water helps you to determine where your body is in relation to space in addition to offering light resistance. If you want something a little more challenging, you can incorporate sprint work or "rapid fire" into your athletic movements. "Rapid fire" is a term we use to describe throwing as many pitches as possible in 30 seconds: perfect form be damned! You can do "rapid fire" with shots or serves too. With "rapid fire," you are just concentrating on moving your body as quickly as possible, so it is a good time to try to push your limits. Don't go over 30 seconds, though, otherwise your recovery will be a bit longer.

All cross-training should include a warm-up that specifically prepares you *for what you are about to do*. If you are about to try to squat 100 pounds, your warm up should be different than if you are going to do "Energy Systems Development." Remember, doing the same warm-up before every activity is not as effective as specializing. Additionally, your cool down should be specific to the muscles you just worked or the muscles that may already be tight. Any good trainer knows this and should be helpful in this area. Remember, your recovery starts the moment you finish your workout. This is true from a nutritional standpoint as well as a physical standpoint.

CHAPTER TEN:
SHOULD I FIRE MY COACH?

Having good mechanics prevents injury and promotes fluid movement and better speed. On a daily basis, I see so many athletes that are not reaching full potential because former coaches gave them misinformation about mechanics or neglected to really perfect their athletic movements. This is your body we're talking about here! I feel like nothing upsets me more than seeing an athlete complaining of an injury that I know could have been prevented if her athletic motion was being executed properly. So here are some things to do and look for in your mechanics, but also things to keep in mind when looking for a coach or personal trainer so that you can get the most out of your training.

First and foremost, to get the most out of your mechanics and get a good idea of where you are already strong versus where you need to improve, you should start keeping a video diary of your athletic movements on your computer. For example, if you are a golfer, you should have someone take video footage of you from every angle (even if it is just on your phone) and place it in a file in your computer. Every month or two, do it again. This would be even better if you have an App like "Coaches' Eye" or "Ubersense" that allows you to slow down or speed up the movements you filmed and draw lines on the images. This makes it so much easier to determine if you are properly aligned with your target.

There are several reasons why keeping a video diary is an essential part of perfecting the movements that your sport requires of you:

1. **You become familiarized with your own athletic motion and its idiosyncrasies**. If you can see yourself constantly pulling your left side out as a hitter for example, you know that is your tendency and you can work to correct it. Over the course of your life, between high school, travel, college, and post-college, you will have many different coaches and they will probably all have different opinions about what makes you successful. If you can see for yourself what you do when you are at your best versus what you do when you are at your worst, you are better able to adjust and be your own best coach.

2. **You should constantly be seeing progress**. Everyone has ups and downs throughout an athletic career, but overall, you should be seeing yourself constantly make little adjustments and improving little bit by little bit. If you don't see progress over a series of several months, ask yourself "why?" Have you really maxed out or do you need to switch coaches? Maybe you need different cross-training or better recovery habits. Maybe you have inhibition or a lack of flexibility in some areas. These are things that a video diary will help you determine.

3. **You will see yourself at your best and worst**. If you are having a rough day, film it and compare it to the best day you have ever had. What are the differences? How can you make good adjustments?

Though all athletic motions have unique biomechanical attributes, most good athletic motions have certain things in common. Here are some simple things to keep in mind when we discuss good mechanics:

1. Everyone is built a little differently. Some people have a higher center of gravity. Some athletes have dense, compact muscles, and others are sinewy and lean. Your feet might pronate slightly while another athlete's might supinate. Make sure that you make minor adjustments for your athletic motion according to your build. For

example, athletes with a higher center of gravity tend to have to work more on core stability. Some athletes who have a valgus twist in the elbow tend to throw more sidearm and therefore really need to be monitored. Your coach should be willing to make slight modifications and not force you into a position that your body cannot tolerate. If your coach refuses to accommodate you, find a new one.

2. Don't ever lock your joints. For example, in the softball pitching motion, it is vital for athletes to learn to straighten the land leg at the right time, but never to lock the joint. Anyone telling you to lock your joint in your motion does not have your safety in mind. Locking joints is something that can really stress the joint, especially when done repetitively.

3. Don't strike on your heel. As a runner, everyone should be looking to create strike on the mid-foot to forefoot. Heel striking in general can leave you susceptible to shin splints and other discomfort.

4. Create the most efficient movement possible. Don't go for flare. You want to get direct to the ball or to the target. If your windup is crooked or offline, you will start compensating in other ways and potentially leave yourself at risk for injury.

5. Train your proprioceptors. Proprioceptors are a class of receptors that are in charge of determining things such as body position and body movement. Proprioceptors are found in the joints, muscles, tendons and inner ear. Proprioceptors enable athletes to maintain balance, determine how and where their bodies are moving in space, and help to prevent muscles from stretching to a point of injury. Proprioceptors are part of a system that helps the peripheral nervous system communicate with the central nervous system. Once the communication has occurred, the central nervous system can interpret the information and provide the body with instructions on how to react. Proprioceptors are damaged when athletes are injured and are typically not fully functioning until well after the tissue has healed. This explains why athletes are often cleared to play and supposedly "recovered" from injuries and yet cannot do the movements they once did so well. Since proprioceptors are so important on so many levels, we should work to train them in our practices. Training the proprioceptors

[50] Laskowski, Edward R., Newcomer-Aney, and Smith. 1997. Refining Rehabilitation With Proprioception Training: Expediting Return to Play. *The Physician and Sports Medicine*.

properly can produce better awareness of space, decreased risk of injury, and better strength. In fact, training the proprioceptors has already been shown to reduce ACL injuries among soccer players.[50] A great way to train and improve proprioception is through use of props. For example, if I see an athlete making an inefficient athletic motion, I will put a pool noodle in the area that is out of alignment. When she hits it, she knows she is incorrect. I also often have my athlete try a movement with her eyes closed and then ask where the body is in relation to space. This allows each athlete to "feel" where she is and what her body is doing.

6. Do the movement slowly and perfectly at first and then gradually speed it up, so that you are promoting perfect practice and good myelination. If you don't know what myelination is, it means you have not yet read *The Talent Code*. Read it, already! If you want a simple explanation of how practice works to make you a superstar, go to http://thetalentcode.com/myelin and you will see. Athletic motions involve a lot of visual processing and physical action. These are things that very specialized areas of the brain deal with. A process called myelination takes place in the white matter of the brain when you practice a specialized movement. Using the same pathways or connections in the brain makes cells wrap layers of myelin around the axons in the brain. As more myelin is wrapped, the signals become faster and more precise, allowing us to perform complex tasks faster and better. The catch, as far as I am concerned, is that these movements really need to be perfect as you practice, otherwise, you are building myelin down the road to distress instead of the road to success. That is why it is crucial that you find the right coach/trainer, which is what we will discuss next.

So now that you know some ways that you can better coach yourself, you might be wondering how to find a really good quality person to help you out with all the other stuff. What does your coach need to do for you? As far as I am concerned, a coach should be doing a lot.

1. At a young age, a coach should be stressing form before winning. I have witnessed some really insane coaches that start screaming at athletes at the 10 and under level. This is a person who is not mentally well. If you are in this situation, change teams, and look for a coach who wants to develop 10 and under players instead of destroy them.

2. Your coach should consider your unique circumstances and not just look as your situation/motion as if it is her own. For example, some hitters can hit really well with bad mechanics but these mechanics cannot be applied to the general population with success. If your coach was great at his or her sport but did some funky things with mechanics, make sure that you are not getting exposed to a technique that might hurt you.

3. Your coach should be a mentor to you. Good instructors know how to relate to people on a personal level. They care about you. They want you to succeed. They wouldn't do anything untoward. Ever. Your coach or instructor should be someone you aspire to be like: not just as an athlete, but also as a person.

4. Some coaches analyze mechanics and others just stick to a philosophy no matter what. This is silly. So many athletes come to me from other coaches who "wanted to change everything." Unless you have had absolutely zero success in the past or are executing mechanics that can really hurt you, there is no need for a coach to go changing everything. These are coaches who want everyone to fit a specific mechanical philosophy without considering little things like success and confidence.

5. Your coach should push you when you need to be pushed, but comfort you when are down and out.

6. Your coach should understand that things are not always mechanical: sometimes problems are more rhythmic. For example, if you are a rower, you might be doing the movements of rowing well, but if your rhythm is not right, you might be wasting valuable energy. Make sure that rhythm is one of the things that your instructor/coach evaluates.

Perhaps you have tried several coaches and you still feel like you are not able to do the correct movements for your sport. Maybe you feel like you just can't develop a good connection with any coach or instructor. This might simply be because of your learning style. There are three different learning styles, and many people are "combination learners," meaning they learn best when a mix of styles are used to instruct them. Many coaches will talk at you without making any adjustments to your body or filming you. These coaches are merely addressing one learning style (auditory). The following are the different learning styles. Try to determine which one(s) represent you so that you can tell your instructors and they will be better able to accommodate you when they explain something.

Auditory Learners: These are individuals who tend to learn best when things are explained to them verbally. They typically enjoy listening and therefore have pretty good speaking and listening skills. Auditory learners tend to remember names but forget faces. When they are trying to solve a problem, they generally like to talk through it. They enjoy speaking on the phone more than meeting in person or texting. They tend to use language that goes with their learning style: "I hear you."

- How coaches and trainers should accommodate this learning style: They should give clear verbal directions when explaining different movements. They should be willing to spend some time speaking with you about goals and aspirations.

- How you can accommodate this learning style: If you have trouble keeping to a regular practice routine, you can set an alarm telling you when it is time to exercise. It is always good to track your progress in a book, but you might want to use the voice recorder on your phone in addition. Make sure that you speak a date with all of your vocal entries so you can review them and hear your progress. For my auditory learners who are also pitchers, I have them close their eyes and listen to the sound that the ball makes when it spins off their fingers. I also like to have auditory learners pick a song to use to establish tempo in their movements. Sometimes a metronome is even helpful if they are going through the movements slower or faster than what is appropriate (this also helps with problems in athletic movements that are rhythmic).

Visual Learners: These individuals do best when they are able to write things down. They are typically pretty organized and detail-oriented. They like charts and illustrations to help them understand what they are doing. They like to have exercises and movements demonstrated for them and described in detail. They remember faces but forget names. Visual learners have good imaginations. If you describe an activity to them, they will generally take a minute to try to visualize it before responding. They prefer to talk in person as opposed to speaking over the phone. They tend to use language that goes with their learning style: "I see what you mean."

- How coaches and trainers should accommodate this learning style: They should encourage visual learners to keep a notebook to write down goals and aspirations. The notebook should also be used to clarify anything that the athlete found confusing. They might even want to draw some pictures of different movements or cut out pictures of the ideal positioning for these movements. Taking pictures or creating video footage of the athlete doing specific exercises is tremendously helpful, particularly if the athlete is executing the movement improperly and cannot seem to correct it with verbal cues. Coaches and instructors need to be patient with visual learners when describing a motion since visual learners will often pause before engaging in the activity so that they can imagine the action described.

- How you can accommodate this learning style: If there are specific movements that you are supposed to be doing at home, get video footage entailing the correct execution of these movements. Take lots of notes and draw pictures and diagrams to help you understand what you are doing. If you need clarification, a Skype session or a session that occurs in person will be much more productive than just having a conversation over the phone. It is particularly good if you have an app like "Coaches' Eye" or "Ubersense," in which you can slow down or speed up video of your motion. I also like to have these athletes practice in front of a mirror.

Kinesthetic/Tactile Learners: These athletes are generally pretty outgoing and demonstrative. They use a lot of gestures and movements to express themselves and come across as very energetic. They enjoy movement and being active. They also enjoy doing new things. Kinesthetic learners don't retain a lot of what they hear. They have a better memory for things they did as opposed to things they heard. They tend to use language that goes with their learning style: "I feel the difference."

- How coaches and trainers should accommodate this learning style: As long as you are comfortable having your coach or trainer move your body for you, she should do that to demonstrate how to best get into key positions. Kinesthetic learners are very responsive when they can feel what they are doing, so a coach is better off spending less time explaining with a kinesthetic learner and more time doing. New drills and exercises are very appealing to kinesthetic learners since they like to experience new things. I use a lot of props with kinesthetic learners so that they can determine where their bodies are in relation to space. There are many very effective ways to use props to help kinesthetic learners develop good proprioception and better memory of the exercises.

- How you can accommodate this learning style: Learn to use different reference points to help you determine where you are in relation to space. Do some of the movements you are trying to learn without weight and/or without the ball and with your eyes closed. This will accentuate your ability to "feel" what you are doing.

Knowing how an athlete learns can make all the difference when it comes to seeing progress and becoming comfortable and confident with important motions. Make sure that your coach/trainer is aware of this and willing to adjust accordingly.

CHAPTER ELEVEN:
GET MOTIVATED BEFORE IT'S TOO LATE

Motivation plays a key role in the life of a successful athlete. Some athletes are more extrinsically motivated: this means that they will work hard on something only because they expect some kind of reward for their efforts. Awards could be fame, scholarships, or material gains. These athletes are often the ones who practice because they know they should, or because dad tells them to, but not because they want to. Other athletes are intrinsically motivated: this means that they work hard at their sport because they love it, are obsessed with perfecting their movements, and so on. Though both kinds of athletes may be successful to a degree, the intrinsically motivated tend to perform more consistently, have better confidence and less stress. Some athletes might be motivated by a combination of factors, such as a deep love of the sport but also the desire for a scholarship. All of these factors can have a tremendous impact on performance.

So how can you use motivation to take your game to the next level?

I have had the amazing good fortune of being able to talk with some world-class athletes. The trigger (motivation) that sparks their climb to greatness is always something that I ask about. Interestingly, every world-class athlete I have ever asked has been able to explain exactly how he or she went from liking his or her sport to feverishly pursuing excellence. A perfect example began in the 1996 Olympics in Atlanta, Georgia. A young Danielle Henderson went to the games to watch the US Softball Team compete. She was already very talented with a bright career ahead of her. She had already spent endless hours throwing into a wall. But after watching the Olympic Team, something changed. She realized that what she wanted more than anything in life was to compete with those athletes at that level. That motivation enabled her to work relentlessly and, after an award-filled collegiate career, she did go on to become an Olympic Gold Medalist.

Professional Iron-Man Triathlete Brendan Brazier had always liked sports, but felt that he was average "at best." Regardless, he wanted nothing more in the world than to become a professional athlete. He explains that he would have tried "anything" if he thought that it would have made him a better athlete. He worked tirelessly on researching nutrition and different training techniques to get the most out of his practices. He spoke with as many amazing athletes as he could to "learn from their mistakes" and build on his knowledge base. He chose the Ironman because he felt that success was based purely on hard work and not innate talent. When getting hit by a car stopped him from training, he founded Vega and was writing books, so that he could help other athletes benefit from his knowledge and avoid his mistakes.

Wow.

If you are feeling like you could never have that level of obsession with your sport, you are not alone. Many athletes work hard because their parents tell them to or because they want to win a game. Unfortunately, these athletes really don't understand how profound intrinsic motivation is and how much it can impact performance. What I have observed lately is that so many athletes are working exclusively towards the vague ambition of a collegiate scholarship, while not really knowing what that requires. These ambitions oftentimes have a lot to do with pressure from parents to try to ease the financial burden of college. Statistically speaking, these ambitions can also be unrealistic, given the amount of money available for most collegiate programs. Many athletes are after a "full ride" to wear like a trophy around their neck, when the truth of the matter is that "full rides" are few and far between. I also find that athletes who are so singularly focused on getting a collegiate scholarship don't perform as well in college as their potential would allow, since they feel that they have already achieved their ultimate goal once their Letter of Intent is signed.

How can we prevent this from happening? We need intrinsic motivation to break through our plateaus and continue to excel.

In my own experience, I would classify myself as mostly extrinsically motivated until I was about 22. I will never forget, because it was the moment that I met Kaci Clark. Kaci is about 5'4" and was Women's Professional Player of the Year for many years in a row. She had also pitched for UCLA and had been invited to try out for the Olympics. When I watched her throw, I felt like I was enlightened. I always felt like I wouldn't be able to throw beyond a certain level because I wasn't 6'4", but here was petite Kaci throwing 68. Not only that, but she had surgery on her arm and at one point the doctors thought she would never pitch again. That was the fire I needed. From there on I became obsessed with perfect mechanics, nutrition, and psychology to make the perfect athlete. After taking a lesson from Kaci and working obsessively on what she showed me, I gained four miles an hour. I was elated. Ever since then I will read everything I can get my hands on about performance. I talk to doctors, coaches, physical therapists, nutrition experts, and elite athletes alike to get the best information. This is information that I apply to my students and myself. This hunger for knowledge is what inspired me to create my TAP (True Athletic Potential) consulting program. It was what inspired me to write this book.

What you have probably noticed in all of these examples:

1. The athlete's desire is ignited

2. The athlete creates a goal that overtakes everything else is his or her life

3. The athlete finds someone (or several people) who will provide support to actualize this goal (this is where I would come in with consulting).

Though igniting intrinsic motivation can sometimes only happen organically, a very good way for you to increase your chances of finding this within yourself is to find someone who inspires you. This should be someone whom you can constantly look up to and learn from. This doesn't have to be an Olympic or professional athlete (although there is nothing wrong with that). The person whom you want to be like may not even play your sport or be your gender. The people who inspire you might change throughout the years. Maybe you idolized Derek Jeter when you were younger, but as you got older someone with a very successful Division I career took you under his wing. These are healthy mentors that can help you to grow as an athlete. Ask them questions. Be a sponge. Like Brendan says, "learn from their mistakes" as much as their successes so you don't have to make a lot of your own mistakes.

Let your goal become you. Setting specific, measurable, and attainable goals has been shown to consistently enable people to reach much higher standards. This means that you need to be able to know EXACTLY what it is that you want to do and then find out the best way to do it. Make sure that there is a way to measure your progress. Keep track of your advancements both mentally and physically. Are you working out because your coach told you to? Or are you working out because there is nothing that you desire more than to push your own limits?

When I first got back from Hofstra camp (after sleeping 14 hours), I went down into my parent's basement with a bucket of sidewalk chalk. I wrote all over the foundation wall that would become my haven for practicing over the next several years. I wrote things like "look the part, act the part, and someday you might be the part" (a favorite Hofstra saying). I absolutely covered that wall with motivational quotes. I was so enthusiastic that I actually made my parents cover it with a sheet when my friends came over. I was embarrassed about how determined I was to become better at pitching and was afraid that my friends wouldn't think it was cool.

In retrospect, if your friends don't think that your desire to succeed is really cool, then they probably won't go very far in life anyway. That is probably a sign that you need some new friends.

With this in mind, are you really getting the most out of your practice? If you are extrinsically motivated, then you might not be concentrating on every serve and every backhand the way you should be. When you run, are you really pushing yourself as hard as you can, or are you just looking at what everyone else is doing?

There is a really big difference between being the best in your age group versus being the best that *you* can be. If you're happy being the best in your school or your age bracket, then you are complacent. Being complacent and not working hard makes it easy for other people to eventually surpass you. If you are really that good, play up. Never settle for just getting out there and smoking everyone in weak competition. To be the best, always compete against the best. It's okay to get humbled every once in a while. That is how you become stronger mentally and physically.

Ask yourself the hard questions today. What is REALLY motivating you and will that allow you to achieve your best potential? Be honest and dig deep. This could be what has been holding you back all along.

CHAPTER TWELVE:
THE MATTER OF MIND OVER MATTER

All athletes go through phases where they may feel like they have hit a wall. In previous chapters, we discussed how this might be related to overtraining, nutrition, improper recovery, motivation, and hydration. Sometimes, however, there is more to it than that. Hitting a mental wall is one of the scariest things that athletes go through because it is one of the hardest things to recover from.

I find myself personally playing the role of psychologist very often as a performance consultant. The mental component of the game has way more to do with consistency than the physical component. I will sometimes have an athlete come in for lessons who has good form but looks like she can't break a pane of glass. When describing her performance in games, she will consistently emphasize her successes over her failures and will therefore continue to build positive experiences. This athlete inevitably gets a reputation as one of those pitchers whom hitters just can't seem to figure out. On the opposite end of the spectrum, I sometimes have an athlete who is a pure stud in lessons, but reports minimal or inconsistent success in game situations. She can't seem to put it all together outside of the lesson.

Why does this happen? A lot of parents out there are quick to respond, "it's confidence!" but to me, this is oversimplifying a very complex problem. Here are some factors that may be contributing:

Focus: Sometimes the athletes who are focused in lessons with feedback coming from only one source (i.e. the instructor) are overwhelmed by stimuli in a game situation. In a game, athletes are dealing with coaches, teammates, the other team, stressful situations, and so forth. Understandably, some athletes have trouble focusing on the task at hand with all of the additional variables. Have you ever noticed how many great athletes describe themselves in game situations as being unable to see, hear, or discern anything outside their immediate goal? Other athletes are just the opposite. They see everything BUT the primary goal. These are often the same athletes who are distracted by a new person entering or leaving a room during lessons or a car driving by. The solution? Work focus like a muscle. We do a drill where the pitcher has to show she is focusing on the catcher's glove in the following manner: the catcher holds up a number with her fingers in front of her glove in the middle of a pitch, and the pitcher has to tell the catcher what that number was at the end of the pitch. You can also gradually and purposefully increase levels of distraction during a lesson thereby encouraging the athlete to focus under increasingly difficult circumstances all the time. I also think that athletes who struggle with focus should try a small group lesson (as opposed to a completely private lesson). In a small group, the athlete is not monitored and given feedback on every single movement. This gives her time to make her own adjustments and also to deal with the distraction of learning and executing athletic movements while other athletes and stimuli are distracting her.

Anxiety: I am slightly taken aback by just how many athletes are nearly paralyzed by anxiety. The 2013 Stress in America survey included teens for the first time and concluded that individuals as young as 13 have unhealthy levels of stress. Athletes this young also really don't understand stress management techniques. Over 30 percent of teens surveyed had felt that their stress levels increased over the past year.[51] In athletics, anxiety is oftentimes triggered by something very simple such as throwing a ball away or having a bad game. Sometimes, it is more complex and clearly a product of the pressure of choosing a college, overzealous parents, or being berated

---

[51] (2014 June). American Teens and Stress. IDEA Fitness Journal. 11(6), 74.

by a coach. Sometimes it is the product of a prolonged illness or injury. An athlete is understandably tentative about playing after a long break, especially if the injury or illness is not completely resolved. This can spiral out of control. Finding the original source of anxiety is essential for correcting this problem. Oftentimes, a sports psychologist or hypnotist can help evaluate the source. Once you are aware of the origination of your anxiety, you can better deal with it. EMDR is another highly effective tool in dealing with anxiety. I personally obtained my certification as a hypnotist after my own mental setback was resolved through hypnosis and EMDR. I have since seen amazing results with my athletes through use of hypnosis. They show improvements in confidence, presence (or "swag"), focus, and relaxation. Yoga and meditation are also highly effective ways of lessening anxiety and improving focus. If you are new to meditation, there are a lot of different types, so find one that is right for you. Meditation has been linked to so many positive things: everything from better overall health to improved focus and decision-making. It would be silly not to use such a powerful tool as an athlete.

Paralysis by Analysis: Do I want you absolutely perfect in a lesson? Yes. That gives you a little latitude in game situations. The truth is that even perfect mechanics will vary somewhat in games as a result of field conditions, the umpire's strike zone, and the batters' preferences. The trick is, you can't obsess over minor imperfections in a game setting. Once you get in the game, you have corrected as much as is possible with your mechanics and you need to focus solely on logistics. If you are a pitcher, this means hitting your spots, evaluating batters for potential weaknesses, and knowing the game situation. If you are thinking about your mechanics on top of all of that, you are not going to be performing optimally. So how do you stop the constant banter in your head telling you to straighten your front leg, snap behind the ball, etc.? It is simple. Understand that kind of critiquing is very valuable, but not when your team needs you. Learn to shift your focus and your awareness to the game and everything that is going on in it. This will eventually overtake your need to constantly self-correct. You cannot undo what happened in the previous pitch and you cannot control what will happen two batters from now. Focus on the present moment only.

Lack of Visualization: The *Journal of Strength and Conditioning Research* published a study showing that experienced competitors who took 30 seconds before their event to imagine their performance did better in both the 10- and the 30-meter sprint.[52] This is what I would refer to as visualization. For pitchers, visualization generally consists of picturing exactly how to execute the perfect pitch and "seeing" where it should go. For a tennis player, visualization would consist of taking a moment to "see" exactly where you want to place your serve. For a basketball player it would be seeing the path to the basket and perfect form for a shot. Once you can visualize something as an athlete, you essentially have a blueprint for doing it in real life. You can spend a long time visualizing, or a very short time (in between serves in a game for example). The point is, if you cannot see yourself achieving your ultimate goals and being successful, the likelihood of that happening is practically non-existent. Take a movement that has been challenging to you and try visualizing your perfect execution of it. You will find that it becomes easier. Practice that as a method for overcoming challenges. Most of the great athletes of our time use visualization on some level to help direct their efforts.

Composure/Attitude: Everyone knows at least one athlete whose attitude has gotten in the way of his or her success. I think pitchers have the worst reputation in this department. A stud athlete might have a very nasty habit of throwing tantrums on the mound. Not only is this a major deterrent for potential recruiters, but also very selfish behavior that is distracting to teammates. I do definitely see this behavior more in "daddy ball." The best way to overcome this obstacle is to determine what triggers it and eliminate those variables immediately. For example, many pitchers lose composure or get an attitude because they are actually angry with

---

[52] (2014 June). Psyching up before a sprint. IDEA Fitness Journal. 11(6). 75.

themselves. If an athlete learns a better way to channel that anger or eliminate it entirely, the problem will resolve. Other athletes simply "lose it" when things aren't going their way. For these athletes, I would suggest creating practice situations where you simulate things not going your way and learn different coping mechanisms. It is a shame to throw away amazing potential because of a lack of composure or bad attitude. Dig deep and find out what the problem really is: it's either that or your career.

You Don't Practice Like You Play: It amazes me how often athletes fail to create competitive situations in practice. If you practice with no pressure on you at all and everyone telling you how great you are, how can you expect to excel when the pressure is on and everyone is yelling at you? In games, adrenaline and cortisol are typically released (that is why you feel so different when competing: hormones are released). Some people do better under these circumstances and some people do worse, but the fact is that if you don't create competition (even if it is just against a friend or teammate), how can you adjust in a game situation?

Your Environment Is Toxic (Team Atmosphere): I have heard so many horror stories about coaches, particularly at the collegiate level, so I understand that being in the wrong environment can destroy you as an athlete and sometimes even as a person. In fact, I am so passionate about this topic that my next book will focus exclusively on it. People were outraged by what happened at Rutgers, but most Division I collegiate athletes could share similar stories. Don't get me wrong, there are some amazing college and travel coaches out there, but you have to find them. If your coach's philosophy involves destroying you mentally or working you so hard that it borders on physically abusive, get out immediately. There is no reason whatsoever for you to stay in an environment like that at any level of play. You can definitely be successful elsewhere.

You Don't Build on Past Successes: Every mistake is crushing. Your confidence is fragile. You are the type of person who can have 10 great games and 1 bad game and you will always dwell on the bad one. Great athletes need to have short memories. Mistakes will always happen, but you have to let them go in order to be able to succeed in sports or in life. If you need to, write down all of the great things you have accomplished in your sport. Read it every time you feel like you want to quit. Fill up an entire book with past successes, no matter how small they may seem, and use it as a reminder of how amazing you can really be. If you are still dwelling on past mistakes, you can write those down too, but then shred those pages or burn them. Learn from your mistakes, but then let them go.

Finally, with any of the aforementioned issues, don't be afraid to ask for help. I have absolutely amazing parents who have always stood in as psychologists for me, but not everyone is so lucky. Even with my amazing support system, I knew when my performance needed the help of a certified professional. A sports psychologist, a behavioral psychologist, a hypnotist or even a social worker are all good options. You should never feel alone when you are going through something difficult. Just make sure that your chosen professional is used to working with athletes and preferably has expertise in your sport. Don't let mental obstacles limit your true potential.

CHAPTER THIRTEEN:
WHEN *TODDLERS AND TIARAS* SEEMS TAME . . .

Over the years, it has come to my attention that athletes' relationships with their parents can be quite complex (read: bat#@%* crazy). In some cases, I think that the moms on *Toddlers and Tiaras* have nothing on a softball mom (and I think we all know who would win in a fight). All kidding aside, though, parents of athletes can be similar to *Toddlers and Tiaras* parents in the sense that both sets of parents coach their child from a young age. It can be really hard after years of doing this to know when to pull back, when to come on strong, and when to let go completely.

When I decided to begin playing softball, my parents' philosophy was "we will match your effort." This is generally a very sound approach. What it meant was that if I practiced a ton then that would earn me the privilege of going to a softball camp or taking a private pitching lesson. If I wanted to practice, Dad would stop whatever he was doing and catch for me or hit me ground balls and fly balls. If I was injured, they would take me to the chiropractor, physical therapist, or anyone they thought would help. To me, this is a very healthy approach. On the other side of that, there are many parents who really push their kids to take lessons when it is clear that the athlete has no interest in ever practicing. This is a waste of everyone's time and money. My dad did *remind* me to practice a little as I got older, but he really only dragged me out there once or twice.

Dad was always really positive about whatever happened in games, even if I didn't do well. He waited until after the game was over to coach me or he would coach me during the times when we practiced together. I loved the fact that he came to almost all of my games. His presence during games always made me confident. We would always talk about batters and game situations in the car on the way home. We would strategize about how to be most effective against the best hitters. "Next game," he would say, "you are facing Deanna Dovak. No matter what, don't let her beat you. Don't give in." We would then proceed to discuss different strategies to work that line up.

Mom only lasted an inning or two at my games before she went to the car. She was too nervous to watch me perform in such high-pressure situations. I think she tried to warm me up pitching once when I was 11 and it bordered on disastrous. Despite that, she supported me in totally different ways. She would always make sure that I had an extra snack before games and remind me to bring the music I liked to psych me up before games. Most importantly, when I was completely overwhelmed and at the breaking point with softball and school, she was clutch emotional support. She even drove all the way into the Bronx one Friday afternoon after I had a particularly rough week.

But she never coached me at all, nor would I expect her to.

Despite all my parents' support and kindness, I always seemed to do better with coaches who were really hard on me and pushed me to my limit. I am still that way. I don't take getting yelled at in an athletic environment as a personal affront. I see it as someone who believes in me and wants to push me to be better. I never saw teachers who marked up my papers and said, "you could do better," as bad guys. I saw them as people who wanted me to achieve my full potential. I worked really hard to please the people that said I stunk the most! I am really grateful for that, especially since, if I really felt like a failure then I knew I could always count on my parents to encourage me to prove any naysayers wrong.

I realize that a lot of athletes are not like me in this regard, and so I don't typically yell at my athletes.

Something that parents have to remember is that, in college, parents are definitely not allowed any input at all. You would probably be amazed at how many athletes actually find this a relief (although I found it kind of difficult at first). Many athletes are afraid to tell their parents that they are ready to approach the sport without constant correction and coaching from a parent. I can understand that you don't want to hurt your parents' feelings, but you *have to speak up*! If mom or dad makes you nervous at lessons or games or puts more pressure on you because you are trying so hard to please them, then you must make them aware. I can't tell you how many hypnosis sessions I have done where a central theme was a fear of "letting dad down." This is not healthy and it definitely detracts from performance.

On the other side of that, there are athletes who are entirely dependent on their parents for mechanical corrections, emotional support and game-time advice. These are typically the girls whose dad has also been their travel coach for their entire lives. These kids often have a love/hate relationship with their parents. It is really hard to shut off your instincts as a parent to make good coaching decisions. It can make life very complicated. These same athletes generally have a really hard time when it comes to transitioning into high school and college. This is understandable, since these athletes have never known any coach other than their parents. It is almost like taking a home-schooled child and putting her into public school for the first time. There is definitely going to be some kicking and screaming going on.

So how can parents strike a reasonable balance? You want to push your child, but you don't want to scar them. You want to be supportive, but you don't want to baby them either (read the letter from my parents at the end of this chapter for good advice).

Well, I will tell you how I found the right balance as an instructor.

When I first started giving lessons, I went to a lot of games. When the girls noticed me there, they would literally look at me every pitch. At first, I used to yell out little adjustments and encouragements, but I found that actually worked very badly. The girls got way too focused on me and it took their focus away from the game. Plus, the travel coaches (understandably) hated when I did that. They don't like to feel as though you are trying to coach over them.

Flash forward several years and I took the opposite approach. I started SNEAKING into games and then telling the girls afterwards that I saw them throw. If they had any questions about their performance, we discussed in between games or during their next lesson. That was better, but it didn't work great either.

Finally, I decided to do the following, which seems to work the best:

-If I planned on going to a game, I usually told the athlete beforehand. Some athletes do not want their instructor at a game because it would increase their nervousness or make them self-conscious. If that was the case, I acknowledged their wishes and didn't go to the game.

-I typically said "hello" to my athlete before the game or I would give her a small wave. I would wait until after the game if my greeting would potentially disrupt the pre-game warm-up or any aspect of the game.

-I would tell my athlete that no matter what I am supporting her but I won't be correcting her at all during the game (so don't look at me!). I told her to keep her focus on the game no matter what and to dig deep for the answers instead of looking to me for them.

-I would tell her not to worry about throwing even several bad pitches in a row because sometimes it takes a little while to get a rhythm or adjust to the umpire's zone.

-I would tell her that she can talk to me in between innings ONLY if she feels like she is really struggling and ONLY IF her coach says it is okay. Otherwise, we will talk after. Some coaches do not want any outside input during games and I think that is completely reasonable. You have to respect that.

I think this is sort of a perfect approach for a parent. This might mean that you have to watch the game from further away for a while, which is okay! I know when I first started having some All-County pitchers playing some top-level games, I did a lot of pacing and biting my lip to keep my mouth shut. That's okay. You are learning new habits, which can often be difficult.

Letting the varsity/college/travel ball coach have complete control in game situations is important, even if you don't agree with their techniques. It is part of letting your child grow up. You can still scout the teams you are playing ahead of time and discuss strategies with your daughter at the dinner table. You can discuss how to react to different scenarios like when curve isn't working, the umpire is not calling an inside pitch or when the other pitcher has a devastating riser. If it's not distracting to her or the team, you can film some pitches or at-bats on your phone. Play it for her the day AFTER the game so SHE can evaluate what she is doing well and what she is doing poorly. Don't tell her what she is doing. Let her push herself to improve and become more self-aware.

It can be really hard to let go of coaching your daughter full-time. That is understandable. You have to remember, though, at some point your daughter will have to fight her own battles (whether it is on the field, in the workplace, or in class). You will always love and support her, but give her a chance to impress you with all that she already knows.

Since I am of the opinion that my parents did an amazing job with regard to sports, academics, and everything in between, below is a letter from them to parents of athletes (if you don't play softball or baseball, the advice is still applicable, just replace "softball" with "basketball" or your primary sport). Additionally, if you are the parent of a college-bound athlete, dad suggests looking at www.payscale.com/college-education-value to get an idea of how much your child's education will be worth when he or she graduates.

Bonus: A letter from Julie's parents

"From Julie's Parents to Your Ears"

If you're reading this the chances are pretty good that you and your daughter have begun a journey down "the road less traveled": a path that will take you into the challenging, exciting, and demanding world of the competitive student athlete. The irony is that, at this critical point in the child's development, you will probably be making important decisions without the benefit of wisdom guided by experience. The reason is simple. There just aren't many people whose own life choices qualify them to offer you some kind of guidance. With that in mind, we thought it might be helpful to share some thoughts, feelings, and insights regarding the life of a student athlete. For the purpose of simplification, we've organized the discussion into three major areas: fastpitch softball, school, and parental involvement.

Fastpitch Softball

First, we have softball. It is a fabulous sport and its popularity is growing in leaps and bounds for good reason. Fastpitch combines strength, speed, agility, teamwork and intellect into a thrilling package that, especially when played and watched at higher levels, is enjoyed by most sports fans and loved by the players and their families.

The centerpiece of game is the pitcher. There is no other team sport that has a position nearly as dominant, and for that reason it is not for the faint of heart. Your daughter has got to *want to pitch*. The very nature of the game puts tremendous pressure on her, and with it comes the inevitability of soaring highs and brutal lows. Perhaps the easiest and healthiest way to measure both you and your daughter's commitment is to simply match her effort. If she is eager to practice, go to lessons, and play, in that order, that's good. If you have to push her, especially to practice, then you may want to keep an option that includes lower expectations.

Whatever the level of play, softball has the ability to teach many valuable life lessons in discipline, resiliency, teamwork, and perspective. For some kids the sport can be a wonderful, recreational experience. For others it can be a stepping stone to a college scholarship. Don't be fooled! Getting a softball scholarship is not nearly as easy as it sounds, even for the very finest players. This would be especially true of someone looking for a "full ride." The fact of the matter is college softball, except in the west and southwest, loses money for the schools. It's not NCAA Football or Basketball, where weekly TV revenues pour in. There is, however, more than one way to earn a scholarship, which brings us to some thoughts on school.

School

The term "student-athlete" should always be used with emphasis added on the word *student*. A good education that prepares youngsters to compete in an ever changing and expanding global marketplace is going to be a whole lot more important than a terrific rise ball.

Basing school-related decisions only on factors connected to softball will likely ruin what needs to be a delicate balance between the two. A student-athlete needs to dedicate a sufficient portion of her time to her homework and to researching prospective, appropriate colleges. Try not to lose sight of the "big picture." Insist that education be kept in proper proportion to athletics. You will be doing your child a great service on two levels. First, she will be forced to efficiently pick her priorities and manage her time accordingly. Second, your daughter will have an opportunity to show the kind of discipline off of the field that has given her such great success on the field. It is important to note that it is just this kind of mix that good colleges find attractive. Good mental discipline equals good pitching.

Remember, we said that schools don't throw (bad pun) a whole lot of money at softball players, but, a young lady who also happens to be a great student gives the recruiting coach an excellent opportunity to plead her case for an academic scholarship. Kids can be eligible for both kinds of grants, or in the case of a school that is not allowed to provide athletic money, a clever coach can help steer the academic money or some campus employment a player's way.

As a rule, Division I schools have the most cash. Division II is next. "D III" programs give no athletic scholarships at all. If you're considering "D I" institutions make sure you and your daughter take a long, hard, even cynical look during any official visits because this will be a commitment spanning her four years in college. She'd better be comfortable with the coach and the girls, because they will be her adopted family throughout her playing career.

Good schools also require freshmen players to attend supervised "study sessions" until an acceptable GPA is established. It is quite possible that your daughter will achieve higher grades in college than she ever has before. Give her a chance here by encouraging her to study hard in high school and prepare well for the SATs and ACTs.

Parental Involvement

One of the most crucial roles of a mom and dad is to monitor the physical, emotional, and mental well-being of their child. It is surely the case when your child is playing the most demanding position in softball.

While fastpitch is a more natural throwing motion than is overhand, the need for proper form is paramount in order to protect the pitcher's body. There is an irresponsible myth, fueled by televised Olympic, college, and professional games, promoting the idea that this motion allows girls to "throw all day." That is dangerous nonsense. Remember, the athletes on your screen have access to individual coaches and a training staff focused on keeping these talented young women in top condition and perfect form. A young girl throwing too many innings can tire, come out of her motion, and hurt herself. Girls who are forced to throw like that at an early age risk damaging their pitching career, or worse, their body.

As tough as it can be to keep good mechanics, it can be even tougher to stay poised and think clearly throughout the course of an important game, a big tournament, or a long softball season. Kids will generally follow their parents lead. If Mom or Dad loses composure, the daughter may at best be embarrassed, or, at worst, follow suit.

These kinds of concerns can be less of a threat if parents properly assess coaches and teams. A program that is a good fit will make the commitment a more enjoyable experience. **Please, never lose sight of the fact that it is supposed to be fun!**

To that end, here are six simple suggestions:

1) When picking a travel team, be careful to choose a program where the coaches have a reputation for being fair, especially if their daughters play the same position as your daughter. As the girls get older teams will be scouted and things can get plenty testy if the players or their families think they're being treated unfairly.

2) Don't go screaming at the umpires. Your daughter doesn't need an angry relative in the stands and you don't want her to lose focus and think the umpire is a bigger threat than the opposing team.

3) It is very important to stay positive while your girl is pitching. A girl's antenna will pick up the slightest sign of anger or frustration, so hide these emotions until there is an appropriate time for their release.

4) It may be difficult, but respect your daughter's decision if she says she doesn't want to be "instructed" during the game. If you see a flaw hold the thought and discuss it when she's ready.

5) Celebrate wins with appropriate gusto, and comfort losses with the proper perspective.

6) Softball pitchers, like many high profile athletes, can receive adulation that is as disproportionate as it is intoxicating. Emphasize remaining humble and grounded. It will not only gain your daughter long term respect but will help her better manage, not only the "ups and downs" of her sport, but, more importantly the highs and lows that await in "the real world."

Finally☺

So there it is. You have the ramblings of parents who, along with their wonderful daughter, have taken a road less traveled. It wasn't easy. If it was, everyone would do it. But there are few things in life more enjoyable and satisfying than watching your child, flush with the confidence and character typical of a successful student athlete, accept, and overcome the challenges presented both on the softball field and in life.

CHAPTER FOURTEEN:
DON'T FALL VICTIM TO TRAVEL WOES AND BORING EATING

As an athlete, you are going to be doing a lot of traveling. Spending time on the road presents many challenges since it alters your eating and your sleep patterns. You will not have all of the amenities you have at home. You will have to eat out at the same terrible places that your team eats at. Very often these places offer mostly "food products" (read: industrialized crap) as opposed to actual food.

Here are some tips to help you along the way:

-**Pack good snacks that will help you to stay alkaline and recover faster**: You must bring whole food snacks that you have tried in the past and that have been proven to work for you. I personally think that there is no better performance line than the Vega Products and they come in travel sizes, so they are really easy to pack. I am not endorsed or sponsored by Vega in any way, even though I have written them like a zillion times, so you know this is really coming from the heart. I always pack Vega Performance Protein, bars, Recovery Accelerator, and endurance products whenever I travel. I also always keep at least a few packets of their electrolytes on hand. In fact, more often than not, if you run into me on the street and ask me for a packet of electrolytes, I can probably oblige. I also recommend packing some nuts and seeds. Find a brand of kale chips/dehydrated vegetables that you really love and pack those. Your hotel rooms won't always have refrigerators (sometimes when you are traveling, the hotel might not even have clean sheets for goodness sake!). Pack some fruits like apples and oranges that travel well without perishing. I also love to pack seaweed snacks, but you know, they are an acquired taste (i.e. Rob said he would only eat them if starving on a desert island).

-**Pack tools to help loosen, massage, and otherwise pamper your muscles**: Of course, you need your uniform and equipment. I also always recommend packing extra underwear and socks (this is just from years and years of travel ball experience). There are some other small things that you can pack that will help you to prep your muscles properly and expedite healing. Obviously, you can't go around traveling with a huge foam roller and most of the facilities you travel to will not have them. However, there is a smaller alternative. When I am coaching, I always bring a Tiger Tail (www.tigertailusa.com) and a small handball for loosening the fascia and working on sore or tender areas. If you know that you are very prone to soreness on the second day of competition, you might want to bring some Epsom salts to soak in the hotel bathtub with after your first day of competition. I recommend packing heating pads that are activated when you open them since these are great for warming up tight areas while you are in the hotel before the game. They are even good for using in the car or bus on the way to the game. If you play a sport that involves gripping the ball in cold weather, these little gems are great to keep with you throughout the game to promote circulation and prevent you from "cooling down" when you don't want to. If you have a specific area where you are experiencing discomfort, have a professional show you how to properly tape it with KT Tape. Make sure that you do this several hours before a game, so that it doesn't peel off when you start to sweat. A lot of people now use compression sleeves or wraps, and these are good for areas that are a source of continued discomfort. They are also easier to apply than KT Tape, and you don't have to worry about them peeling off. On the other side of that, it is not nearly as specific as KT Tape or Kinesio Tape, and therefore might not address your specific needs. If you are prone to pain, you might want to also pack some arnica and/or turmeric (check with your healthcare provider). Know where you can get ice at all times since you will undoubtedly need it after you are done for the day. You probably want to pack a yoga band to help you stretch after games. I also always recommend packing a good quality probiotic and/or digestive enzymes like the kind made by Healthforce Naturals (again, not sponsored by them, I just think their products are the best), because traveling and playing competitively can sometimes make butterflies in your stomach. Also, if you are playing in a foreign country (as will often be the case with really competitive athletes) there are different strains of bacteria in the foods and it is grown in different soil. This can sometimes lead to digestive upset and you want to be prepared.

-**Pack music/motivational tools**: I always used to listen to ridiculous, crazy, screamy music to get me psyched up before games. I am the type of person who needs to be alone so that I can focus and get serious. Many athletes need other things to help motivate and inspire them before games, however, such as inspiring quotes, videos, notes from other players and so on. If you have had success with hypnosis in the past, you might want to get a CD made for you of a hypnosis session to relax you and focus you before games. Know what works for you and make sure that you always have it with you to help you perform optimally.

-**Use Yelp**: If you type "vegan restaurants" or "organic restaurants" or even "vegetarian restaurants" into Yelp, it will come up with a bunch of different options near your current location. Most ethnic foods are pretty friendly towards plant-based eaters, so Mexican (as long as the beans aren't cooked in lard), Indian, Japanese, Thai or Ethiopian are all good options. Just always ask for your Thai food without the fish sauce. I recognize that you will probably not be the most popular person on the team if you suggest eating at an ethnic place every single meal. On a recent trip, however, the coach I was traveling with (read: my softball mentor) did think it was a good experience to get all of the girls to try Ethiopian. I would say that all but two really enjoyed it and it made my night since Ethiopian is pretty much my favorite ethnic food ever. Even if ethnic food is not your thing, though, you can use Yelp to look at different menus and see where they have the best salads and freshest vegetables. My go-to meal if I am stuck in a place that has absolutely no vegan options is a huge plate of either steamed or grilled veggies. This is usually not on the menu, but most restaurants are happy to oblige, especially if you ask nicely. Throw some nuts, salt, and maybe avocado on there and you have a good post-competition meal (again, broccoli is not the best thing for pre-competition).

-What if your team only eats at fastfood chains and Wawa?

Then you need to hire me to come speak for them or buy several copies of this book. All kidding aside, though, most teams do tend to eat this way because it is cheap and fast. If you are eating at a place like Panera, it is a bit easier because you can get black bean soup and they will make any of the salads there without the meat. If your team is all into McDonald's however, that is a tough spot. I think you can really only ever get oatmeal, fruit or salad there, and even then, only in emergency situations since most of their "food" is genetically modified and/or sprayed with chemicals that should probably be illegal. 7-11 or Wawa both have some good choices. You can always get nuts and fruits there. Plus, you can usually get some containers of chopped carrots and celery or tomatoes and cucumbers. 7-11 and/or Wawa also usually have green tea, which is a good source of antioxidants and energy (it does have caffeine). Planet Smoothie now has plant-based protein and about a million options that involve some really yummy fruits and vegetables. A smoothie is a great way to cool down after a tough workout. They even have a green smoothie now, which I have had multiple times and it is delicious. It's a great way to get some greens in without tasting like you are getting greens in. Starbucks now has a salad that is basically vegetables and brown rice.

It tastes really good and only takes about 2 seconds to purchase. Starbucks sometimes also has seasonal fruits. If you are lucky enough to be in an area where they have a "Juice Press" or similar store, you can pretty much just close your eyes and pick anything and it is all pretty good for you. These stores are becoming very common in New York City (thankfully). It is basically organic, plant-based, raw fast food. Can we say, "best idea ever?" I think so.

-**How to get your sleep on**: If you take yourself seriously as an athlete, you probably want to choke the people whom you are assigned to room with when they are up all night or leave the television on or start blasting music at 1 am. These things and worse happen in a collegiate environment, especially if your coach is not good about enforcing a curfew. When I was doing travel ball in high school, my dad always got a room with an extra bed or a pull out sofa so that I could sleep in his room if the girls I was assigned to got too crazy. This is not an option for many people, which is unfortunate, since you need to be well-rested to perform your best and much of your recovery and muscle building happens when you sleep. Prepare yourself for loud roommates by packing earplugs and a sleeping mask. I know it doesn't make you look super cool, but sometimes it is the only option if you are bunking in one room with three other athletes that don't care about their performance. If you think that these are extreme steps to take, here is a direct quote from an INR seminar I attended on "Food, Stress, and the Brain":

> When we expose our bodies to light, food and activity at times when our organs and cells expect dark, quiet and sleep instead, it can cause desynchrony or misalignment of our natural circadian clocks . . .In humans, even brief circadian misalignment results in adverse metabolic change (eg change in appetite hormones, inflammation and insulin resistance) and cardiovascular consequences.[53]

---

[53] INR: "Food, Stress, and the Brain"

If you are groggy when waking up in the morning before games (read: me), expose yourself to bright lights in the morning. If you have trouble sleeping on the road, use the following guidelines:

1. Avoid bright light before you go to bed.
2. Try to finish eating 2-3 hours before bed.
3. Wind down and avoid electronics before bed.
4. Try to go to bed and wake up at the same time every day.
5. Have a bedtime ritual that will signal your body that it is time to go to bed.[54]
6. Consider packing chamomile tea for your trips. It is very calming before bed (NEVER recommended before a performance). It is great for promoting sleep at the right time, especially if you just changed time zones.

Other tips:

-Learn about different fruits and vegetables, especially superfoods. There are entire books dedicated to superfoods, and I could write a bunch just about those, but that is for another time. A lot of people are concerned that when they switch to a plant-based diet (or primarily plant-based diet) they won't have anything to eat or they will be eating the same things over and over. Others insist that they don't like fruits and vegetables but then again, most people think corn is a vegetable (it is technically a grain). There are so many options and unique preparations that "I don't like fruits and vegetables" just doesn't fly. Below is a list of fruits, vegetables, mushrooms, nuts, seeds, pseudograins and grains to get you started (the superfoods are starred). This list is by no means exhaustive, and all of these foods can have unique and exciting preparations (particularly the sea vegetables and mushrooms), so do a little research and find the ones that you enjoy the most.

[54] http://sleepfoundation.org/sleep-tools-tips/healthy-sleep-tips

Fruits

Acai*

Apples

Apricots

Bananas

Blueberries

Cantaloupe

Cherries

Coconut

Dragonfruit*

Figs

Goji Berries*

Gooseberries

Grapes

Honeydew Melon

Kiwis

Lucuma*

Lychee

Macquai*

Mamey Sapote

Mangosteen

Mulberries*

Nectarines

Oranges

Peaches

Pears

Pineapples

Rambutan

Watermelons

Green Vegetables

Arugula

Broccoli

Collard Greens

Kale

Mustard Greens

Purslane

Romaine

Spinach

Swiss Chard

Watercress

Sea Algae

Chlorella

Spirulina

Sea Vegetables

Arame

Dulse

Hijiki

Kelp

Kombu

Nori

Sea beans

Wakame

Root Vegetables

Beets

Black Salsify

Burdock Root

Carrots

Celeriac

Ginger

Jicama

Maca*

Potatoes

Parsnips

Radish

Tiger Nuts*

Turnips

Yucca

Squash (there are lots of other varieties of squash, so see what is local and fresh)

Acorn squash

Butternut Squash (great for soup!)

Pumpkins

Spaghetti Squash

Zucchini

Other Vegetables

Artichoke

Asparagus

Brussels sprouts

Cabbage

Celery

Eggplant

Fennel

Green Beans

Jerusalem Artichokes

Leeks

Okra

Onions

Tomatoes

Mushrooms

Black Trumpet

Button

Chanterelles

Chicken of the Woods

Cremini

Maitake

Oyster

Porcini

Portobello

Reishi*

Shiitake

Truffles

Nuts

Almonds

Brazil Nuts

Cashews

Chestnuts

Hazelnuts

Macadamia Nuts

Pecans

Pili Nuts

Pine Nuts

Pistachios

Walnuts

Seeds

Chia Seeds

Flax Seeds

Hemp Seeds

Pumpkin Seeds

Sesame Seeds

Sunflower Seeds

Pseudograins

Amaranth

Buckwheat

Quinoa

Grains

Barley

Bulgur

Corn

Farro

Kamut

Millet

Oats

Rice (brown, red, or "forbidden rice")

Sorghum

Teff

Wheat (try to eat only minimally processed or "sprouted wheat" products)

Make food exciting by trying new spices and new preparations all of the time. Your body will get lots of great protection from these foods and your palate will be enlightened.

Finally, here is a little "cheat sheet" I developed to help you understand how to be at your best throughout the day of your performance:

Pre-Game:

- **Hydration**: At least two cups of water a half hour prior to getting on the field

- **Nutrition**: Complex carbs plus good fats (especially Omega 3s)

- **Example:** Buckwheat pancakes with berries and almond butter.

- **Why**: Most people consume too many Omega 6s, which can contribute to inflammation in excess. Omega 3 fats balance them out. Good quality carbs (like pseudograins and fruit) provide your body with fuel, as does *good quality* fat (no donuts!).

- **Activity**: Heat anything that may be tight from the previous day prior to rolling. Roll out any tight areas prior to dynamic stretching. Some areas to consider are: back, traps, ribs, pec minor, medial deltoid, forearm, biceps, triceps, quads, hamstrings, IT band, calves.

- **Why**: Rolling flattens the fascia and loosens up any tight areas, making injury less likely.

During Competition/Between Games:

- **Hydration**: Water is absorbed best during the early stages of activity, so you should be drinking a lot at that time. Heavy sweaters should consume electrolytes early on, and everyone else should start consuming them an hour after activity. Vega makes some great electrolytes, but so does Ultima http://ultimareplenisher.com/

- **Nutrition:** You wouldn't need to eat during a game, but could use a gel if you felt like you were bonking. If you are an endurance athlete, you might need to pack some snacks that won't be difficult to digest. If you are looking for something in between games, it would be similar to the nutritional profile of what you eat pre-game.

- **Examples of in-between game nutrition**: Almond butter and jelly on sprouted whole wheat or brown rice bread, Vega endurance bar, fruits and nuts, coconut oil.

- **Why**: You are still looking for foods to help you with energy and stamina. You also need things that are very easy to digest, and protein is not the easiest thing to digest quickly.

Immediately Post Competition:

- **Hydration:** This is where I personally drink an absurd amount of water, but hydration depends somewhat on weather, sweat loss, and activity level. Athletes just need to keep in mind that if they are drinking a ton of water they do want to keep putting in electrolytes occasionally because otherwise the electrolytes become diluted and can actually contribute to fatigue.

- **Nutrition**: Eat a 4:1 carbohydrate to protein ratio to replenish depleted glycogen stores within 30-45 minutes of completed competition. You do not want to take in much more than 10 grams of protein during this time as it may interfere with your body's ability to stay hydrated.

- **Example**: I like seaweed or Kale chips, but I realize that most athletes will not be too into that. A great combo is some cacao nibs with goji berries (about a handful is good) since that provides all nine essential amino acids and a ton of antioxidants.

- **Why**: Regardless of what kind of activity you perform, you will have depleted glycogen when you finish if it was an intense workout

- **Activity**: Cool down, static stretch, recovery pose (see the website for pictures), ice

Post Competition (usually about 2 hours after the game):

- **Hydration**: Hydrate as needed, but hydrate more if you are even mildly sunburned

- **Nutrition**: This is the best time to take in a ton of green vegetables and protein. Remember, don't eat too much more than 26 grams of protein in a sitting (more can be stored as fat or be taxing to your internal organs). Stick to around 60 grams of carbs (less is okay at this point, if you would prefer).

- **Example**: The mushroom recipe on my Youtube page is a good one if consumed with a leafy green salad. This is a great time for quinoa, rice and beans, spinach, broccoli, kale, etc. Stay away from things like dairy and soda.

- **Why**: The protein will help repair damaged tissue and the plant-based foods will help restore alkalinity and promote recovery.

- **Activity**: You can do recovery pose, or you can pulse hot and cold on any uncomfortable areas. You can do an Epsom salt bath. I am personally too tall for my bathtub at home, so I have to kind of squirm around and soak one area at a time. If you are tall, you might experience a similar situation in a hotel bathroom, so plan on soaking the areas that need it the most. If you have already showered and don't plan on showering again before the game the next day, this is an excellent time to do some KT taping or Kinesio taping (depending on what is available). The more sleep you get the faster you will recover.

Though this book contains a ton of information, it all works best when customized to yourself or your team. I recognize that much of this information can be difficult to understand at first and is always better when explained in person. For help with this, the best thing to do is a consultation or seminar. Even if you choose not to do either of these, however, I recommend filling out the following form so that you have a lot of information about your habits, strengths, and weaknesses.

Form For Private Consultation

Name:

Age:

Phone Number:

Email:

Sport:

Primary goal:

Nutrition

Please fill out the following for at least 3 days. Try to notice how you feel in the hours following what you consume (i.e. full, tired, energized, etc.). Include beverages and times of meals and snacks. Be as specific as possible (you can keep a journal instead, if preferred). Also try to note what specifically you eat prior to your workout/game, during your workout/game, and after:

	Day One	Day Two	Day Three
Breakfast			
Snack			
Lunch			
Snack			
Dinner			

Why types of vitamins and/or supplements (include brands) do you take and why?

Do you have any known allergies or food sensitivities?

What prescription medications do you take?

Do you have any major health concerns?

Injury/ Training

How often do you workout/practice? What is typically the duration of your workout?

How do you warm up prior to a game or workout?

What types of workouts do you do and on what days (make a calendar or keep a notebook if preferred)?

Do you set goals for each of your workouts/practice sessions? If so, what specifically are you working on?

What types of injuries have you incurred?

How have you treated injuries in the past?

Rest/ Recovery

What do you do to recover after practice/working out?

How many hours of sleep do you get a night?

Do you have a specific routine before you go to bed?

Do you frequently wake up in the middle of the night and/or have difficulty falling asleep?

Psychological

What do you do to mentally prepare for a game and how soon before a game does this begin?

What was the worst athletic performance of your life?

What was the best athletic performance of your life?

Do you tend to perform better in a game or in practice?

Do you suffer from any compulsive tendencies? If so, please explain:

Do you frequently experience anxiety? If so, please explain:

How do you generally get along with your teammates? What is usually your role on the team?

Focus

How would your describe your ability to focus?

Is focus heightened or worsened in game situations?

What are situations that you find distracting (or things that you know diminish your focus)?

ABOUT THE AUTHOR

Julianne is a sports performance consultant and a certified personal trainer. She has studied nutrition, kinematics, performance and recovery. She became a certified hypnotist several years ago to help her athletes overcome mental barriers. She has produced countless All-County athletes and dozens of successful collegiate athletes. She was part of the coaching staff that took LIU Post to the College World Series in 2011. She was a four-time Academic All-American and Valedictorian of her college graduating class, even though an injury nearly destroyed her career. Julianne has spent the last ten years developing her True Athletic Potential (TAP) Program. It is a program designed to allow athletes of all levels to maximize their abilities. It was nothing short of an obsession that involved interviewing some of the best coaches, athletic trainers, therapists, nutritionists and social workers that the industry has to offer. She is available for group/team lectures, seminars, and consultations.

Contact: juliannesoviero@gmail.com

(631) 737-0196

www.trueathleticpotential.com

www.flawlessfastpitch.com

For more gorgeous images like you see on the cover, visit Kristina Strobel's website at http://www.kristinastrobel.com

Made in the USA
Middletown, DE
14 February 2022

61177880R00106